The Way Home

By the same author

I Close My Eyes and See

published by Findhorn Press

The Way Home

Chronicles of an Inner Journey

by
Dorothy Lewis

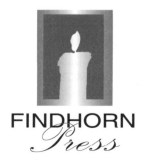

FINDHORN
Press

British Library Cataloguing-in-Publication Data.
A catalogue record for this book is available from
the British Library.

Set in Palatino by Findhorn Press
Cover illustration and design by Posthouse Printing

Printed and bound by Interprint Ltd, Malta

Published by
Findhorn Press
The Park, Findhorn
Forres IV36 0TZ
Scotland
tel +44 (0)1309 690582/fax 690036
e-mail thierry@findhorn.org
http://www.gaia.org/findhornpress/ *or*
http://www.mcn.org/findhorn/press/

Contents

Introduction

Sometimes, travelling on the inner journey, I have felt very alone. I used to think this made good sense. We are born alone and we die alone, so it is only to be expected that as we forge our life path, between the birth and death gates, this also must be a solitary task.

From time to time, however, we do meet other travellers. Some have travelled further, and longer, than we have. Some are at the beginning of the journey. Some are at a similar stage to ourselves. We share the similarities, note the differences, encourage and are encouraged, get new ideas, and find we are links in a huge network of travellers.

And at what surprising places we happen to meet! Waiting at the railway station, standing in a supermarket queue, even through a sentence which leaps out of a book scanned quickly in a bookshop. There are face to face conversations occasionally, yes — but once our antennae are tuned and alert, we may recognise another traveller just through a quick eye contact, a cheery remark, a passing touch of comfort.

These contacts have always been to me a source of strength and encouragement, a reminder that in spite of difficulties — environment, health, age — travel persistently continues all around the planet. The inner journey flourishes.

I am telling here the story of a very ordinary woman. No fame, no wealth, little material advantage. But over the last twenty years an increasing awareness of the inner journey has provided for her a different quality of richness. This, like all richness, must be shared. Shadows too, for naturally these deepen as Light increases. And the Life lessons, coming thick and fast — and sometimes needing to be repeated when they are not learned. All are to be shared, and in the sharing to offer a further recognition, with comfort, love and trust. For I have found that the Life Flow is always waiting to carry you safely, if you can just *allow*. It sounds so easy — it can feel so difficult.

And there is more. Sometimes as I struggle through an arid patch in my journey, a dry and desolate desert, I become aware that other travellers, unseen, are in the same place. Maybe we can meet, openly, at the next oasis? By contrast, as joy flourishes and I need to foster its flow by passing it on, it almost feels as though we are dancing, all of us together — a vast and wonderful circle dance on top of a mountain somewhere.

So I am not alone. The occasional outer meetings always bring sustenance. When they are missing I can still hear, if I listen carefully, some of the thousands and thousands of footsteps of my unseen travelling companions. Like me, they are finding their own way home.

Chapter One

My name is Dorothy. I am nearing 70 and I am a traveller. Or should I say an explorer? What have I explored? What do I explore now? Am I too old? Is it time to stop, for old age, and wait quietly to die? No way. Dying, after all, is only another aspect of living and I shall continue to learn, explore, discover, right up to the death gate, and I expect way beyond. Maybe my outer activities will need to be curtailed, but the inner journey is not in time or space. As I get older it stretches still — away and away and away, as well as within and within and within.

Looking back I see how much my outer journey has reflected this need to push on. Through my life I have moved house many times, been married, raised children, changed jobs, and shared a wide variety of relationships. In earlier days certainly I submitted to the conventional role of wife and mother — I washed, ironed, cleaned, changed the beds, polished the windows, mended, cooked, gardened, washed scraped knees, bandaged broken heads . . .

And I sometimes wonder what would have become of me if our marriage had survived? Would I now still be quietly cleaning, cooking, mending, gardening? Without children, filling the long hours with coffee mornings, whist drives, Mills and Boon, endless knitting? Perhaps not. Perhaps the new life had to break through.

Outside, I have never travelled far, being content with quiet seaside holidays, country B&B, simple days out in beautiful places. I have had no money for far travel, but no real desire either. Inside . . . ah, that is different. And these are the explorations I need to share with you, as I reach a stage in life that offers greater space.

For life seems to offer such clearly defined stages: a

daughter at home, then an independent young woman, then a partnership, children, career, and finally old age. What a lot to learn at each stage, about space and timing. As a child the necessity, often overplayed, of fitting into someone else's pattern. "Hurry up." "Stop daydreaming." "Go and do your homework." Then leaving home, discovering a truly individual space, sometimes the first experience of real aloneness and self-organisation. Maybe learning, too, the conflicts of shared adulthood, with peers, in house, bedsit, college room. Then the closer joy and conflict of shared partner space. And eventually the huge space of the retired life and status of OAP.

There are all sorts of ways of filling space. Many of us at any and each life stage tend to do this frenetically, unwilling to meet ourselves in the surrounding emptiness. But now I am able to use some of this freedom to stop and look back. Not to hold on, or regret, but to see when and what I learned, in those outer travels, about myself, about life. And to notice how in some life stages there seemed no time for anything but the job in hand. Where was 'I' at those times?

All unwittingly, I think I was adding insight, experience, extension to my constricted life-start. The inner exploration had begun. And I believe that it is through the inner exploration that meaning, purpose, love and trust have evolved, running threadlike through the outer hustle and bustle. Each time a new stage evolved this woman, like all the others, had to adjust, and each time the inner growing quietly continued.

My outer life, till now, has been busy busy. When my marriage broke I had an income to earn and four children still to rear. There had to be a major change. As a mature student I trained as a teacher, while we staggered on, on a wing and a prayer. And yet, looking back, it was amazing how Life supported me.

We found a cottage that was tiny but adequate. Because

the dear old lady who was selling it liked me, she knocked the price right down. After only four years of teaching, my boss dared me to apply for a wonderful job — Head of Infants at a brand new school, open plan, team-teaching. It was all outside my experience, so I treated the interview as a huge joke and nearly backed away in stark fear when I was appointed.

From there I eventually took a year out to do a Dip.Ed., but in order to proceed to an M.Ed. I needed money. Tongue in cheek, I approached the local College of Education, saying I was of good worth and needed a lectureship for a year before doing a Master's degree. Again, I was stunned to be accepted. Looking back from here I can see and understand that somehow I had become immersed in the stream of the Life Flow, and was being carried. We'll talk about that later.

It was only when the fourth child left home that my Inner Life really came to the surface and could be recognised. From that time, twenty years ago, I have travelled and explored, had some wonderful times, and occasionally fallen flat on my face. In desperate times it has been hard to meditate or travel the journey consciously, but always there has been a sense of some sort of remaining *inner* security.

So what happened outwardly when this new energy surfaced? Well, it was a another time of complete outer change, with new home and new lifestyle. I almost felt as though I was being pushed, and yet, paradoxically, being freed. I think perhaps for the first time I jumped out of safety, out of the reasonable, and followed my intuition. For 25 years I had been almost entirely occupied with meeting other people's needs. Not an unhappy time, in the main. I loved being with children, and found teaching and lecturing really creative.

But suddenly I was on my own. At that time there was a great cutback in Colleges of Education. My particular

College was closing, so I was going to have to apply for jobs elsewhere. And I realised that to gain promotion I would almost certainly have to move into a city.

Somewhere inside me a small voice said, "Why do you want promotion? What will you gain?" And the only answer I could think of was more money. "What are you going to spend the money on? Clothes, holidays . . . ?" And then that persistent little voice asked, "What would you most like to do, now you are on your own?"

And I had no doubt. I have always felt at home in the country, the wilder the better. To live there was my real dream, and I had found the actual place one summer a few years earlier. The children, bless them, had ganged up on me and said, "Mum, you *must* have a holiday. The girls, 18 and 16, looked after the boys, 14 and 12, with a kind neighbour as failsafe, and I drove away in my little Mini to explore the Yorkshire Dales "for as long as my money holds out" . . .

And it lasted. The first B&B, hearing my story, took me in hand. At breakfast the wife came in and with her back to the rest of the guests whispered, "My husband says this should last you all day." Such a plate of bacon, eggs, sausages, mushrooms you have never seen. I waded through it and he was right. I stayed there three days, then moved on. And again fate looked on me kindly.

I visited a little church in Wensleydale, just as the cleaning lady was busily mopping and polishing. "Do you know of anyone who does B&B?" She stopped, leaned on her mop and regarded me intently. I almost felt I was being undressed. "*I* take people, if I like the look of them." There was a long silence. Finally I dared ask, "Would I be all right?"

She was wonderful, a real Dales character. The cottage was spotless and the cost incredibly low because, as she apologetically explained, "The lavatory is outside, I'm afraid, but there is a chamber pot in your room, for night time." And there it was, indeed, large and comfortable, and spattered profusely with roses. On the Sunday evening I decided to splash out on an 'evening meal'. (Usually I just heated beans or soup on my Gaz stove). Her face fell. "Oh dear," she said, "I can't do a proper evening meal on a Sunday because of church. I could do you just a High Tea about five, if that would do."

It would do. Apart from the two enormous fresh-laid boiled eggs the table groaned with every sort of Yorkshire baking. She hovered over me, offering more tea, more butter, more jam, more . . . And then, just as I finished, there was a huge clap of thunder.

My little lady almost literally turned pale green. "I daren't go to church in a thunderstorm," she wailed. "Oh dear, oh dear." It was my turn. "You'll be perfectly all right with me," I declared boldly. "I'll take you over to the church and pop you right inside. Get your coat on. We'll be off." Clutching me desperately she obeyed, and all was well.

Finally I finished with Wensleydale, and as I crossed the Buttertubs Pass into Swaledale it seemed as though my soul stirred and said, "This is where you belong." I drove into Reeth, and the huge green, held within the hills, surrounded by little stone houses, seemed to bid me welcome. This was the place of my dream.

So, five years later, the immediate nonsensical answer to "What would you like to do most?" was "I'd like to live in Swaledale." I did try to be sensible. Still with one College term left I asked my children if they had plans for Christmas. Reassured, I booked a cottage in Reeth over Christmas and New Year. To try it out in winter.

I still remember that time as magic. I had a ridiculous tiny Yorkshire terrier pup with me, and we walked endlessly, and sometimes played — I remember chasing her in the heather, in the moonlight. Each day, as it got dark, I came in to my comfortable cottage, cooked a hearty meal, and relaxed with knitting, TV and books. On Christmas Day I packed a picnic and went up high on Fremington Edge in the cold sunshine. Half way up I was startled to hear Christmas Carols floating up from the village. The village band was making its annual tour. The best Christmas. And I *knew* I needed to live there.

I was right, because it just happened. I decided to apply to the North Riding for an ordinary Assistant Teacher's job, and then look for a house. I asked the cottage owner to look out for one for me, and he said, "What about the house on the green?" "Not *now!*" But I had a look anyway, and the builder came, on Christmas Eve, to cost the needed renovations.

I had enough money to last till the summer, and I had my M.Ed. thesis to write, as easily there as anywhere — another term to finish the preparatory research. But it was a mad leap in the dark, and I couldn't understand the intuitive certainty that it was right.

As soon as I got home I rang a friend who was an estate agent and asked him to come and value my bungalow near Hull. I had no idea what it was worth. Bought in 1970 it had cost only £4,500, but now, in 1976, there was a housing boom. I needed £12,000 in all.

Jim came over and spent what seemed like years looking round, up in the loft, tapping woodwork, examining wiring and plumbing. Finally he appeared. I deliberately hadn't told him what was needed. "What could I get then?" I asked. "I would suggest a straight twelve thousand," was his reply. Two weeks later it was sold, to a young couple who were marrying in May. So in April I moved to a borrowed cottage in Wensleydale, and the builders moved into the Reeth cottage.

I can't believe it was all just 'luck'. I *needed* to trust an intuitive move. I needed to uncover so much of myself that had been lying hidden for nearly fifty years. I needed, too, to find a place in the outer world that could reflect and be nourished by my inner journeying. And, from then on, what a journey!

The magic continued. Quite casually, it seemed, I was housed again, for the duration of the Reeth alterations. Attending a committee meeting at a Quaker school and chatting to the staff, I mentioned my impending move. "Oh," said the Art staff, "we've got a cottage in Wensleydale. Would you like to use it till you can move in?"

I had a wonderful few months there. I laid out all my thesis material, undisturbed, on their vast dining room table, and licked it steadily into shape, visiting Reeth two or three times a week to check on the progress of the house. In between, small dog and I walked miles in the surrounding countryside.

At last it was done, and I moved in. But no job appeared! I hadn't known I was going to leave teaching as well. Would I have dared to move if I had? I did get a few supply places, and for the whole of the autumn term I replaced an Infant Teacher away on a course — the total Infant Department consisted of nine children.

What next? Lateral thinking. As the Spring came I decided to turn my house into a tiny guest house. I could offer three bedrooms and a guest sitting room, although only one bathroom and loo. The house was right on the green. Views from the front were lovely, but the view from the loo, overlooking the fell, was magnificent.

For the first season I put a brief advert in *The Dalesman*, but most of my guests came from an advertisement in the Quaker magazine, *The Friend*. 'Held in the hand of the hollow of the hills, tiny guest house offers welcome.' With hindsight I realise that this was a 'given' message. I certainly didn't sit down and think it out. Guests came back as many as three times a season. As word spread, the season lengthened, March to November, but in spite of earnest pleas I refused to open for Christmas.

Although I could only take six guests, singlehanded it

was hard work. I learned the hard way. Most people booked for dinner, bed and breakfast, and I soon discovered the most successful menus. It fascinated me how many people, even in the early 80s, were not familiar with good simple home-cooking, away from the frying pan. Shepherd's pie was a favourite. The men's eyes lit up at the sight of treacle sponge. Timing was the worst bit — everything hot and ready at the right moment. I learned to provide only one complicated dish. A fussy dessert was preceded by a casserole, a joint with all trimmings followed by something from the fridge. Homemade soups were perhaps the main draw. Little did the guests know how some were concocted. I remember one evening when I served a new recipe as vegetable: leeks in sage sauce. Everyone took a polite spoonful, but most of it was returned to the kitchen. Out came the blender, and a little more stock, and next day: "What *lovely* soup, what *did* you put in it?" Aha.

There were baddies too, alas recommended by a Quaker family. A psychotic woman found an imagined slight and attacked me. Trapped in the front porch, behind the sturdy front door, I really thought my end had come. Icily calm, I heard myself say, "If it's so bad, why don't you get the police?" It worked. She frogmarched me to the kitchen, heaved the whole phone fitment off the wall, and after phoning retired, all sweetness and light, to the guest sitting-room, to charm the local policeman. This didn't work, and in a very short time the family was on its way. I was so shaken that the week following, when a male guest unexpectedly came out of the sitting room as I was locking up, I screamed! Horrified, he asked why, and I told the story. Next day as guests came back from their day out I was presented with not one but two gorgeous bouquets of gladioli, as comfort.

On the whole, I met lovely, lovely people. The little old lady, well into her eighties, who asked if I would mind giving her a lift up to the moors, she would *so* like to dance in the heather! My favourite couple, both vastly over-weight, walked all day, ate a substantial dinner, and after a little socialising retired early to bed. There, each night, they demolished between them a large box of chocolates as they read. Many coast-to-coast walkers used Reeth for a welcome mid-walk pause. They came into the village about three o'clock, left their muddy boots in the stone-flagged hall, and wearily climbed the stairs to their room. "The water's hot, how about a bath? Would you like a cup of tea? Run the bath and I'll bring it up." They were ideal guests — cup of tea in the bath, lie out on the bed till dinner time, and in bed again before ten.

It was a good three years. I so enjoyed the different people, meeting their various needs, showing interest in their life happenings when they wanted to share. And they often did. Looking back, I think a really strong energy of love and caring built up in the house. And of course it was reciprocal. Great tension for everyone when the tiny Yorkshire pups were imminent, and utter delight at the mouselike safe deliveries. One guest commented, "Your animals are always so friendly. You can always tell what people are like by their animals!"

So what happened to my newly opening inner life in all this busyness? Was it lost, or ignored? No. In these three years there was so much sharing, for guests were safe enough in a warm and comfortable country place to be truly vulnerable. I learned about other people's beliefs and trust. Many Quakers came, and went over the fell to Meeting in Wensleydale. Many others had no apparent religious belief, but found something up on the moors that to them was 'other' and renewing. I respected this as a spiritual link — different but no less of worth than that of those who needed a formal pattern to their spirituality.

One set of guests were keen Mormons — lovely people who agonisingly prayed for my deliverance, hell-bound because not of their fold. I tried to explain that I could totally respect their beliefs as right for them, but expected the same respect for me and mine. It felt extraordinary to be assured that the type of healing I was using was of the devil. I looked them straight in the eye and said, "You know me well now. Can you honestly believe I am practising something evil?" Quite genuinely and in sadness they replied, "Ah, but the devil is cunning. You can easily be duped." It was unanswerable, and eventually our friendship had to close.

My life at that time was sharply divided. Summer was crammed full of people and events, winter was a beautiful private space. Time then for *me* — to walk on the moor, sit quietly at the window looking out at the green, read, study, listen to music, and explore new openings. And they came.

It seemed that my first commitment to following intuitive direction — moving to Reeth, trusting, and changing my lifestyle, started a steady process that has never stopped. As far as I can, I live in the *now,* and people and events continue to turn up at the 'right' time.

The next happening scared me stiff. I awoke one morning to find that the fells suddenly looked like cardboard theatre props. My head and reason told me quite clearly that if I walked up there, the ground would be as usual, and I would walk over into the next valley. But my eyes told me they were not 'real', could almost be lifted up and put away.

I didn't understand this and found it very scary. I avoided looking up at scenery. Dogwalks were down by the river, or through the fields. For several weeks I kept getting the same impression, until one day I visited my daughter, some forty miles away across the Pennines. Driving back I suddenly felt extraordinarily tired. I turned off the main road into a little lane, took a rug from the car, found a sheltered place in a field and stretched out, with the little dog, for a nap.

When I awoke I was quite cold, and found I had been there for several hours. To my delighted surprise everything was back to normal. I could climb the fells again.

What was happening? I think now that I was actually moving into a different stage of awareness. What I was seeing, or being shown, was a first glimpse of the difference between inner reality and outer unreality. We so much believe in our material surroundings as being all there is, all of life. We collect possessions, compete and struggle to achieve materially, and yet . . . ? The really 'best' things in our lives can *not* be seen — love, harmlessness, joy, relationship. Non-material, very precious, very real, very spiritual.

That was the first happening. The second came from a Christmas present — a book on leylines and dowsing, from one of my nephews. This was quite new to me. I had never heard of energy lines and, perhaps surprisingly, had never heard of dowsing either, a practice of finding water by holding twigs that move as the dowser crosses an underground stream. It can be used to find energy lines, too, and lost property, maybe even lost people. It all sounded a bit weird, but as it was winter and I wasn't busy I made some experimental 'rods' out of wire coathangers, as suggested, and followed the diagrams at the back of the book. Could I do it? To my surprise, I could. And I tried using a pendulum too, a weight on a string, swinging it back and forth till it gyrated.

I wasn't really sure if I was imagining it. Books from the library led me to more experiments, and finally I wrote to the British Society of Dowsers and asked if there was an experienced dowser anywhere near at hand who could check me out.

The result was a wonderful afternoon visit to a farm near Consett, and a lovely man who took me out into the fields to experiment. First he gave me some very good

advice: "Ignore all the tarrydiddle written about dowsing. It's a natural sense you're using. Forget about facing
West, and taking deep breaths, never wearing rubber
shoes, all the silly 'rules' ignorant folk concoct. You've got
your wellies. Put them on, and let's get on out."

He himself used a small pair of whalebone rods, bound
together at one end. But although he showed me how to
hold them, they seemed too tightly sprung for me to manage. So he broke off two hazel twigs and still I got no result.
(I know *now* that, first, I was holding them far too tightly
in my nervousness and, second, I was firmly telling
myself I couldn't do it — a self-fulfilling prophecy!)

That day I watched in amazement as he strode across
the field, rods dipping as he entered the stream's energy,
dipping again as he left it. From the distance between the
two, he could calculate the depth. But I couldn't do it.
Disappointing. Suddenly I wondered,"Is there any way
you can do this using a pendulum?" "Oh yes. It will gyrate
one way as you go on, and another as you come off. It's
just more difficult if there's a strong wind."

I had been experimenting at home with this and that,
and one of my daughters had given me an old-fashioned
heavy brass plumb line, for outside use, hung on a piece
of binder twine. "You'll have to go in a different field." So
we crossed over to the next field, and he opened the gate,
saying, "Right, off you go." It looked enormous, this great
stretch of land ahead of me, and I quailed. But I was determined to try, and strode off, swinging the plumb line as I
went. I was amazed when it suddenly started gyrating to
the right. I kept walking and after nine or ten strides it
gyrated the other way. I looked round. "I'll come and
check you," he called. I held my breath. He crossed the
field as I had, and at the identical places the rods dipped.
"Congratulations," he said. "You're a dowser."

We went inside then, for an amazing farmhouse tea.
He had a fund of stories to tell, as he was in great demand

for his dowsing. Often it was just to find a place to sink a well. But sometimes factories asked him to pinpoint sources of pollution. He said it was really amusing when he arrived at these places. Men had usually been detailed to help him carry his equipment. They stood gaping when he pulled the two small strips of whalebone out of his top pocket.

One factory was in real trouble for polluting a nearby river with its waste material.The owners just could not understand it, as they had gone to considerable trouble to see that the waste was safely buried at a great distance from the river. When my man pulled out his rods and investigated, he found that all unwittingly they had buried it just above an underground stream that fed directly into the river. He told them where it would be safe to dig, and the problem was solved.

He gave me another piece of sound advice. "You need to specialise with your dowsing skill. Use it to find water, or missing people, or lost objects, or in any area that seems best to you. But choose. It is better not to try to be a jack of all trades. I did find my wife's lost wedding ring, and I do use dowsing for the odd domestic job at home. But I decided to specialise in finding water, and I think you'd do well to discover your own special area."

I don't know how I knew, but immediately I felt that for me it must have something to do with healing. And so it has — though I have to confess that I always keep a pendulum in the kitchen drawer ready to sort out the odd cooking query. Is the food fresh? Is the fruitcake cooked? And, ah, the perfect soft-boiled egg, gyration indicating when white is firm and yolk is soft.

So that winter I practised dowsing, in a fairly crude way. At the turn of the year I moved on to the next stage of the journey, 'happening number three' (after which I stopped counting!). A friend asked me to a New Year party. Just chat and drinks, and a lavish buffet supper. So

I drove over to Wensleydale again and mingled with a crowd, mostly strangers, letting their hair down as the New Year came in.

I found myself standing next to a young blonde woman, up from London, and idly asked what her job was. "Oh," she said, "I'm training to be a Transpersonal Psychology counsellor." She was startled when I then began to ask her intelligent questions — the first person she'd encountered who had even a vague idea of what she was talking about. I'd read a relevant article in *The Guardian* just a couple of days before, and had found it interesting. She told me details about the course and the people who ran it, and confirmed that, yes, transpersonal psychology included study not only of the conscious and unconscious, but also the *super*conscious, or transpersonal, or 'other'. Just what I needed?

She promised to send me details of workshops etc. when she got back to London. As with the usual sort of promise made at a party, I didn't expect to hear any more. However, a week later, along came the programme and application forms, and I felt drawn to this new adventure. A twinge of nervousness hit me. The questions asked included: "Have you had any mental illness? We need to know this in relation to the fantasy work." Immediately I wondered how dangerous it might be to travel into the hidden consciousness. Should I go?

Again, I think I was pushed. My new friend offered to put me up for the weekend, my application was accepted, it was the slack season for the guest house. Off I went.

There were about twenty of us, all told. We went round the circle briefly, introducing ourselves. I remember the feeling of awe when one man said he was a healer. I cannot actually remember the theme of that first weekend. I think it was probably simple self-exploration, finding sub-personalities and, inevitably, inner connections.

I loved the fantasising, and then the writing down or

drawing, and the shared experience and code cracking. For all the work came out in symbolism. We had to find the meaning for ourselves. The process was so simple, lying relaxed and comfortable on the floor as we were told a story, allowing our own unconscious to fill in the given gaps, as appropriate to each person.

I wish now that I had kept a record of those early fantasies. I think that they were almost mind-blowing — so simple and yet somehow so able to cut through the outside life clutter and produce material which at the least made me think and at best proved life-changing.

One hugely significant fantasy I remember very clearly from those early days. We were told to get ready, in our imagination, to go on a journey, an heroic journey, and to see ourselves prepared for it. The picture that instantly came to mind was myself as a rather beautiful young knight, clad entirely in shining gold. Entirely, that is, until I looked at my feet. There, in total contrast, was a large pair of very ordinary walking boots. I giggled at the ridiculous picture, then hastily quietened, remembering this was a serious exercise.

We were told to choose three helpful tools to take with us. I found a sturdy staff, and a little old man with a long white beard. The third tool I could not understand at all — it was a very pregnant cow.

Eventually we all came to a cave, and were told to go down into it to find our treasure. I decided I'd better leave the cow up on the surface, so I tied her up there, and the little old man, holding his staff, stayed to look after her.

The entrance to the cave was very dark, and I gingerly felt my way down. After a while it began to get lighter, and finally I came out into the cave and to an amazing sight. Almost the whole of the cave was filled with an enormous multi-faceted crystal. Behind the crystal shone an absolutely brilliant white light — far too bright to look at directly. It shone through the crystal, and every facet was a different colour, and it all hummed with a sort of aliveness.

I just stood looking at this in total awe and wonder and it seemed no time till the story remorselessly continued. "Now, take your treasure and go back up out of the cave." Again I almost laughed. How could I carry that great crystal? And immediately the answer came. "Your job is to create little cats'-eyes of those colours, all over the world."

When I came out of the cave, the little old man was smiling broadly and there, beside the cow, was a brand new tan and white calf. A wonderful end to the story.

There didn't seem to be the need for a great deal of interpretation. The walking boots were to remind me to keep my feet well on the ground as I travelled the inner journey. My job was clearly stated, and within the whole fantasy was the feel of the numinous, the 'other'. Yet this new birth in me, symbolised by the new calf, related also to the outer life.

I returned to Swaledale on the Monday. Next day I took the dogs out for their usual walk. In the corner of one field there was a cow who appeared to be in some sort of difficulty. I put the dogs on the lead and went to investigate. To my amazement, in front of my eyes the cow gave birth to 'my' tan and white calf. This was synchronicity, a reality I experienced time and time again, as did my clients, when inner and outer lives merged. Often it was a signal for new creativity.

Chapter Two

So now I had discovered dowsing and also uncovered a huge delight in colour. I seemed newly sensitised. Life in Swaledale offered wonderful vistas. Green was an endless multiple of shades. Each tree was different. Even the same tree changed through the day, as light moved among the branches. Every season offered new delights. Bracken appeared, fresh green, then dusty green, and finally all sorts of russet shades. After rain, in the autumn, its glowing tan, almost of copper, shone out on the fellside. At the time I didn't realise it, but I think I was already beginning to program my brain computer to produce at a later time exactly what I would need for colour healing. Then, it was just a new pleasure.

The guest house was still my source of income. But I was well aware that it was a stopgap, to be enjoyed as another experience for the 'now'. I started looking for the next outer move, delving into a thick paperback that listed all sorts of New Age occupations — alternative medicine, healing, readings, communities, activities. I was looking for any form of healing that included dowsing and colour. It was an unlikely combination, but these two aspects had impressed me so forcibly.

I found a method called radionics. It sounded extremely way out, something to do with working with energies, adding colour, 'broadcasting' healing vibes. This was all so new. My conventional middle class upbringing, formal religious practice, clear black-and-white morality and, most important, 'sensible' reasoning seemed almost flouted by these new experiences.

I *needed* my walking boots symbol. I used them a good deal for real. On the light summer nights, when guests were fed and watered, I used to go out and walk on the hills. If I was tired I just climbed up and sat, watching the clouds in the sky and the shadows below me, feeling the aliveness and lovely earthiness of the scene. Down by the river I used to chat to the cattle, who shared their warm breath with me.

One afternoon I sat by the river, transfixed, as for half an hour, only yards away, a pair of young kingfishers fished. From their perch on a branch suddenly one would drop like a stone, emerging with a small silver wriggle in its beak, then back up to the branch to relish its meal.

They knew I was there, and I asked, in my mind, if they would like to come closer. I had barely produced the thought when both birds crossed the river and flew past me, only inches from my face. Coming back, they made a draught as they passed behind me. Startled, I said, "Thank you," and they calmly went back to their fishing.

A few minutes later, hikers went by on the far side and the birds flew away. I walked home in a sort of daze. It was like a present of communication, a tiny scrap of life synthesis. The picture is vivid, even years later.

So what about radionics? The best way to suss it out seemed to be to try it, as a patient. So I wrote to the Radionic Association and was given the address of a practitioner sixty miles away. I rang to enquire, and she sent me a sheaf of information and a case sheet to fill in. She also asked for a tiny bit of my hair, to be used as an 'energy focus'. I learned more about this as I went along.

Meanwhile I did as I was asked, and presented for her attention a fairly intractable and long-standing gut problem. I was told that as soon as possible she would do a full 'analysis' of my energy systems, write to report on this, and then treat me for a month, all for the initial fee. I should note that the analysis was not the same as a doctor's diagnosis, as it related entirely to the energy systems so to speak 'behind' the physical presentation.

A very few days later I received a note saying that

unfortunately she would not be able to do the whole analysis before going on holiday, but on a quick look had found evidence of food sensitivity. Would I cut out beef and tomatoes from my diet meanwhile?

The result was good, and for the next 15 years this practitioner very adequately helped me deal with both minor and major health problems. Some years later I had to be hospitalised for major surgery. With radionic support healing was startlingly rapid — I was walking about the ward in a couple of days, standing upright at that. But the best bit for me was to be able to fall into a deep, childlike sleep around 10 pm each night, and sleep through till lights-on at 6 am — this in spite of residual discomfort and the noisy surgical ward.

Tentatively I said I might like to become a practitioner. After talking it over, applying, being interviewed and being allocated a tutor, I embarked on the two-year course. It was home-based, with monthly tutorial visits, a number of weekend seminars, and a steady system of examination.

To describe radionics in full would necessitate a separate chapter, even a whole book. In absolute brief it is a system which teaches subtle anatomy, and also the energy patterns for each organ, tissue, nerve, etc., in perfection. These, through the radionic method, just need affirmation. But there are also energy patterns for the various diseases, and these need correction.

The analysis of the patient's mental, emotional and etheric/physical energies is accomplished by dowsing over the patient's hair sample, neatly anchored between two sticky circles — and labelled! The resulting indications are threefold: percentage of chakra disturbance; over- or underactive flows in the three main energy areas — mental, emotional, etheric; and specific troubled areas as expressed through the physical. Treatment is given by sending to the patient, by means of various instruments, the necessary patterns of affirmation or correction.

Most practitioners have a variety of increasingly sophisticated instruments to help pinpoint the areas in need of attention, and to 'broadcast' the corrective energy patterns. These patterns, incidentally, are translated into sets of figures, known as 'rates', that can be set up and released appropriately. The shock set, for example, is 10.10.4, the correction for inflammation 40. These rates, listed in several fat books, are selected again by dowsing.

While I was training I was still making ends meet by running the guest house, and therefore had little spare cash for instruments. Somehow I discovered that supplementary home-made mock-ups also worked, for me. This, of course, made sense. The real power behind radionics is the power of thought. Practitioners in training gradually learn to focus their thought accurately, and the rates — perhaps because they are used by a large number of people, on the same pattern of thought — are an additional means of focus.

I can't remember how long I had been practising when I discovered that just writing the rates down, with instruction, worked for me, without instruments. I discovered this in an amusing way. A fellow practitioner, who bred German shepherd dogs, brought her mother to see me one day, a fifty or sixty mile drive. When they arrived, she got out of the car looking pale green. They had brought two large pups with them, both of which had had a busy time throwing up in all directions as they travelled.

"*Please* treat them for the journey home," she requested. So I took a snippet of hair from each, put them on the instrument, and gave them appropriate treatments of anti-nausea, and to settle stomach and pylorus. When she got home she rang to say thank-you. All had been well.

But a couple of weeks later she rang again to ask if I had any ideas. She and her husband, complete with dogs, were going on a touring holiday in Scotland. "I can't ring you up every time we decide to move on," she said. "I almost feel I'll have to put them in kennels. But it seems such a shame. They'd love it up there."

And immediately I knew the answer. "I'll write the two treatments down on a postcard for you. Keep it in the front of the car, and each time you move on, clip the hair onto the card to activate it." They had no trouble at all. To me this indicated two things. First, the dogs could not have known what was happening, so it was not just a case of 'mind over matter', wishful thinking and the like. Second, it seemed to give me permission to treat human patients with the same method — that is, just by noting the treatment needed, with time and length of treatment, on the treatment sheet.

This was my way of doing it. My own practitioner used many instruments, and I got the benefit from *her* way. But once again there was affirmation of my dawning belief — even as a student — that the power of focused thought, regardless of surface 'frills', was the real basis of radionic treatment.

The colour part of the treatment also changed for me. Initially, we were given a pack of transparent colour slips. We dowsed for these as well as for the appropriate rates, and they sat on top of the hair sample while treatment was given. As a recipient of treatment I was often aware of the colour my practitioner was using. A deep blue, or a clear yellow, or a warm rose would suddenly come to mind.

But later I found this method too limiting, and instead of using slips I would write down on the treatment sheet, beside the chosen rates, whatever colour came to mind. Perhaps the bright green of early beech leaves, or the deep, dark blue of summer darkness, and so on. And my patients often 'knew' what colours they were receiving. One mother wrote to say that her seven-year-old daughter, my patient for some years, had asked for her bedroom to be painted peach. She had not told her that I had commented that the child always seemed to need peach.

I sometimes think we humans are so insensitive, or perhaps just resistant. My two cats responded readily to treatment. Worms, fleas, ticks departed like magic. Small injuries also cleared up very quickly. One cat was ginger, the other honey, and both inevitably needed a very pretty pale green with their treatment. This made a nice colour scheme. What I hadn't realised was that the cats knew all about it. I was treating patients one morning, and one patient needed that particular green. From nowhere, with a great whirr and purr, the large ginger cat shot into the room, jumped on the table and, purring loudly, sat as near the colourslip as she could get.

But colour with radionics did not seem to me really to be 'laying cats'-eyes all over the world'. That came in a different way. When I started my radionics training there were no tutors in the north of England, so I had to go down to London for my monthly tutorial. And again, in the Life-Flow, I was steered in the right direction.

I found the right address, and a little old lady with grey curly hair and a white overall opened the door to me. This was Lily Cornford, an amazing and wonderful healer. She sat me down at a small table at the side of the room. "Practise on this patient," she directed, giving me a chart and a hair sample. "I'm not quite finished, but I'll be with you shortly." And she returned to the couch in the window to continue with whatever she was doing.

A few minutes later she saw the patient out. "Now, my dear, come and sit down, and we'll get to know each other." We sat opposite each other quietly. She had very beautiful brown eyes, and for what seemed like a very long time she just looked at me. I felt as though several layers were being removed. Finally, "You have such beautiful creative energy. But, oh dear, you have such fixed ideas. We'll have to do something about that." It completely threw me. At the time I didn't realise exactly what she meant. But I felt undoubtedly she was right. And indeed she was.

I asked what she had been doing. "Oh, it was colour healing." I probably looked confused, as I had seen no evidence of lamps, colour slides, and so on. "*Mental* colour healing," she explained. And I heard myself saying, "Will you teach me? I need to use colour."

Over the next two years she taught me a system which I loved, and still use, though in a personally modified way. Half way through my radionics training my own practitioner completed her tutor training, so I transferred to her, then needing only an hour's journey to my monthly sessions. But also once a month, leaving Swaledale early in the morning, and getting back late at night, I travelled to London for my hour with Lily and her colour healing. It was a wonderful day, for I managed also to fit in a visit to Barbara, one of the directors of the Centre for Transpersonal Psychology, for an hour of personal therapy.

While my inner journey was moving on, sometimes almost too fast, my personality energies had a lot of sorting to do. I had been a very lonely, isolated 'afterthought' in a professional family. Then came the war and I was an evacuee in Canada. I always had the feeling of being 'a nuisance', left out, even unwanted. My desire for higher education was unfulfilled, as my parents were old and couldn't finance it — another grievance. So at 21 I leaped into marriage, to be with someone who would love *me*, as of major importance! It was disastrous, in a long drawn out, painful way, and totally reinforced my lack of self-worth.

So my hour in therapy with Barbara, working from a transpersonal viewpoint, helped me to connect with my real inner strength, and to begin to flourish as the person I had been born to be.

And of course, it wasn't all plain sailing. After transferring my radionics training I visited my own practitioner. It felt strange. She was a lovely woman, slightly older than me, living in a vast and wonderful 'county' type house, with a farm on the estate. She thought nothing of entertaining fifty or sixty people in some charity affair, had a close and demanding relationship with her four sons, and supported her husband in his various pursuits. On top of this she had a large radionics practice and tutored trainees. I grew to love her deeply. Whenever I rang up and presented a problem, her motherly voice said comfortingly, "Oh dear, I'm so sorry. Never mind, we'll put it right." And she did.

But, to me then, she presented a total duality: dressed in conventional tweed skirt, sweater and pearls, leaning over a strip of hair with a pendulum in her hand. I came home, my mind reeling and, of course, transferred the doubts to myself.

Was it really the right thing for me to do? *Should* I try to adapt to such a different and as yet unproven lifestyle? Did any of it make sense, or was I just jumping into some sort of deep end before I could swim. Worse, supposing I did jump and then found I could never learn to swim?

Someone suggested that a really good astrology reading might help. My only knowledge of astrology was from bits in the Sunday paper, though I knew there must be more to it than that. However, through the Centre for Transpersonal Psychology, I was introduced to Liz Greene, then an up and coming figure and now of international repute. You needed to send her your date, place and time of birth, and the fee. Then after a few weeks she arranged an appointment in London, and you were asked to bring a two-hour tape to record the conversation.

I was impressed. The first thing she asked was whether I was sure that my birth time was accurate. I assured her it was. "One of my sisters is like the elephant who never forgets. If she said it was 10 am, then 10 am it was."

I told her that I knew nothing about astrology and was not, just then, particularly interested in the theory, which I could read up on later. Would she just interpret? She did this brilliantly and I was fascinated at the way it clarified my attitudes and outlook. Much of the reading indicated my need for the inner search. At that time this made particular sense. She also described my father and mother very accurately, and this was helpful.

But two main aspects really affirmed the current changes in my life. The first was simple information. From the Sunday papers I knew that my sun sign was Libra, the sign of harmony and balance. I think I had always felt fairly guilty that although indeed I worked to those ends, I also seemed to have a very deep and stormy side to my nature. Heavy emotions tended to catch me unaware, and I felt a consistent need to know what was behind a surface situation. When Liz told me that both my ascendant and my moon were in Scorpio, and explained the nature of that sign, it all made sense. It felt as though I had suddenly been given permission to acknowledge the whole of me, instead of just the presenting polite and mediating role. The second aspect came to light when I told her why I had really come — because of the confusion in my life, and uncertainty as to the right decision. *Was* I meant to be moving into the area of healing? Was I the right sort of person?

I shall always remember the way she looked at me and replied, "This has been waiting for you for nearly fifty years. It's more than time you got started!"

At the end of the two hours she said. "Your time of birth was correct. This exactly fits you." I commented that it sounded a difficult patterning. How could air (Libra) and water (Scorpio) be comfortable together? "Don't see it as difficult. See it as a challenge. And remember, this is your birth pattern. It is not set to dominate you, but is for you to use. As you grow, the emphases will change." And they have.

I came home to spend time consolidating the new skills, ideas, beliefs. There were the radionics tutorials and seminars, which gave me a lot of new contacts. There was the monthly visit to London. The guest house kept ticking over, and a few flying visits to Hull enabled me to complete my M.Ed. thesis and send it for binding. It was all go.

But amidst the bustle I found time to meditate and study. Lily had recommended that I start working with the Arcane School, an esoteric spiritual school which was run entirely on correspondence lines. This proved exactly right for me. Study booklets arrived, work was set, and monthly meditation reports had to be sent in. A time factor was suggested, but was not rigid. Some sets of work were meant to last six months, some a year, but one could work more slowly, or sometimes faster, as one's life allowed. The whole system was run on spiritual trust, without stated fees. The responsibility for giving financial support was one's own.

Two tenets were made clear. The first was to do with personal responsibility. The work was suggested, but never chased. Impersonality was encouraged, so after the first year or so one sent one's work to an unspecified group for comment. There was therefore no personal dependence, and comments were impartial, constructive and non-critical. It was suggested that students test the work in their own lives, and only accept what they personally found valid.

The second and more important tenet was that one lived what one studied. There was no space for delving into isolated theory, or 'escaping' into meditation. The work taught about energies and forces, and how to use energies in positive ways, such as through healing. One learned about detachment, and how sometimes to scrutinise one's life — not with any emotional bias, blame or guilt, but rather to watch patterns unfolding, to spot trouble areas, and to begin to change them. And all the while to treat other people with love and respect, while beginning to experience the synthesis that is possible between all life energies.

Sometimes I despaired of *ever* integrating warring personality energies, and of making soul contact. Nevertheless the main aim of the work was not to 'improve' oneself, but to grow in deeper understanding, so as to be available for service in whatever way life presented.

It was like a gentle drip from a tap — no pressure, no persuasion. This is here. Use it if it is for you. Indeed, the course proved self-regulating. Those for whom it was not appropriate just dropped out. For me it was invaluable as a discipline. How could I send in a meditation report if I had not meditated? Over the years I think it has given me a sort of steady backbone to the fluidity of life change that has evolved as I have continued on the inner way.

What next? By now I had completed the radionics training, and was in my probationary year. This meant I could begin to charge a minuscule fee as I worked. I was still under a certain amount of supervision and the final examination/assessment still loomed, prior to my acceptance for full membership of the Radionic Association.

What about healing? Lily kept saying, "Go on, use it. Stop being so proud." For of course it was pride that stopped me. I knew *I* wasn't going to be providing the healing, just acting as the channel for it. But what if nothing happened? What if I made a fool of myself? What if . . . ? From the now of today I can look back with a wry compassion. I was so lacking in trust, so ignorant.

But at last I broke the pride barrier. Many of my radionics patients liked to come for a visit. I included this as an optional within the initial fee. I enjoyed visits. Radionics as a profession can be quite isolating. In the main part contact is by phone or letter and, of course, distances can be enormous. My furthest patient was a small girl in India, thousands of miles away.

On this particular occasion the patient had come from the other side of the Pennines. We talked about the analysis and the initial treatment, had a cup of tea, and then I heard myself saying, "Would you like some colour healing before you go?" She was delighted.

So we went up to the bedroom, as I had not yet acquired a couch, and as she lay comfortably on the bed I carefully followed the routine and pattern of channelling I had been taught. The motive 'for the patient's best good'. The solar plexus protection from any negative energies. The aura cleansing, the deep concentration on colours needed for each energy centre, the final sweep and settling for the patient as I went, symbolically, to wash my hands.

The patient got up looking radiant. She said she felt wonderful and set off happily on the long drive home. I closed the door behind her and immediately a thunderbolt struck me! My head and back just blazed with pain. I couldn't imagine what had gone wrong, but as it persisted I rang my radionics practitioner and said, "Please *do* something."

An hour later it was still as bad, so I rang Lily. "Oh dear," she said in her gentle voice. "Oh dear, I didn't expect this. You have just pulled in too much power. Next time, don't concentrate; just stand back and allow the healing energy to flow through you. Don't worry, I can help you now."

And certainly a few minutes later the pain was gone, leaving me nevertheless somewhat shaken. For very many months after that, when I asked that the healing be for the patient's best good, I quietly added 'and mine'. But it was an effective lesson about the actual power available, and also the danger of ignorant meddling. I also learned that 'you get what you ask for, so be careful what you ask'.

There is a myth going around that you cannot offer healing if you are unwell yourself. This made no sense to me for two reasons. First, the healing is coming through you, not from you, and the energy is whole and radiant. Second, what is 'well'? Must I be perfect, whole, consistently radiant? What human being can reach, much less maintain, this standard? So where is the line drawn? I would not, for simple infective reasons, stand close beside a person if I had 'flu. But if I am below par, then as I start the healing process I ask, "May I receive this too?" And I feel better after sharing a healing session. This, I believe, is how it should be. To be depleted is to 'try' to heal with one's own energy. This may be the way for some people, but not for me.

However, having sorted out that bit of reasoning, I was taken aback by a phone call thanking me for some healing work I had done with the relation of another healer. Genuinely, and without false pride, I commented, "Well, I'm very glad, but it's really nothing to do with me." Back came the blistering reply, "Don't be so stupid, of course it's to do with you. You may be a channel, but do you really think it makes no difference if you're a grubby sewage pipe instead of a clear, clean conduit?"

She was right of course, and I passed this on when I started to run healing workshops. I also felt that I needed to point out, "If you decide to be a healer then, willy-nilly, your life will change."

How does it change, and why? I think the simple answer is that you begin to look at things from a different place. So the bit you see — of a person, an animal, a plant, any life-form, or of a job, a responsibility, a relationship — looks different from this perspective. Killing becomes abhorrent, limitation often unnecessary, openness and vulnerability worthwhile risks, and synthesis a real possibility. Almost, it seems, one's life turns round and spirals off in a different direction. The outer circumstances may appear exactly the same. The inner perception tells you something else. The whole process really means that one begins to live not by seeing the outer and taking it in, but from the Centre and taking it out. Just living inside out, perhaps.

And there is a love affair! A love affair with Life. Like any love affair, it settles down. Humanity remains selfish, forgetful, cruel, sometimes despairing. Duality hits you in the gut. Sometimes it is hard to remember that you have access to inner strength, light and love.

Chapter Three

The concept of love was something I had to relearn. Perhaps it had been one of my entrenched fixed ideas. What love meant to me at that time could be described as caring, watching over, sharing difficulties, touching, holding and most particularly expressed tenderness. So I found it incredibly difficult to think of love as an impersonal energy — an energy I could use in radionics without any personal element. *Dis*passionate love!

The first time this sank in was when I was a recipient of it. One evening, while busy preparing dinner in the guest house, I was suddenly devastated by a phone call from my elder son. His wife had just told him she had met someone else and was leaving him. He was deeply distressed, and when I eventually put the phone down, saying I would ring later, I started to cry myself. Tears dripped into the soup and salted the cabbage, and try as I might I could not turn them off. The situation was doubtless pressing buttons about my own failed marriage.

Finally I rang my radionics practitioner — oh saver-from-disaster — and said, "Please *do* something. I can't serve dinner in this runny state." A few minutes later my head felt as though it had been filled with a sort of soft cotton wool. The tears stopped, and I joked and chatted with the guests as usual, though I felt decidedly odd and detached.

Dinner over, I rang her back. "Thanks very much, you can take it off now. I feel stuffed. And I think I can cope." She laughed. "I only gave you one treatment — love."

The second incident was more dramatic. This time I was the practitioner. Friends of friends had heard of my work and rang to ask if I could help a little Down's syndrome boy. They told me the details. Jimmy was four years old and lived with his Grandma who adored him and dealt with his problems uncomplainingly. He was virtually helpless, doubly incontinent, and could not speak or move unaided. He spent most of his time sitting on the floor in front of a large colour TV. The colour and movement appealed to him. He appeared happy.

Grandma washed him, dressed him, changed him and sat him on the floor. At mealtimes she sat him in a highchair, fed him, changed him again, and so it went on. Sometimes she took him out in his pushchair, and he beamed at everybody before returning to the telly.

I was still fairly new to radionics when I said I would try to help. For a few weeks I gave him just about every treatment in the book. Nothing happened. Then, coming downstairs one morning it seemed as though my intuition shouted at me, "He just needs LOVE, with red." We had been warned in our training that red was a very acute stimulus and should be used with great care. But at this point in the journey I had come to realise that a very clear intuitive insight needs to be trusted, without question.

For ten days that little boy was soaked in the impersonal love energy, transmitted on bright red. A regular rocket of a treatment. And his first ever adventure was almost to set the house on fire!

It was washday. Grandma was in the scullery washing. Clothes were drying round the fire in the kitchen, and Jimmy, as usual, was settled on the living room floor, with toys and telly. Today was to be different, though. For the first time in his life he moved, solo, across the living room floor, through the door, across the passage, into the kitchen, and knocked the clothes horse towards the fire.

Grandma was amazed and delighted. And from that day Jimmy started to respond to the other treatments — brain, limbs, coordination. Gradually, over 18 months, he learned to stand, to walk, to become continent, and finally to be able to attend Special School. I never heard the end of it, as his parents were Mormons, and at this stage decided that healing which was not church blessed was of the devil. But I knew progress would continue. All through 'love'.

It cropped up in the colour healing too. One day a woman came for healing, saying she was continually depressed and struggling, and felt she had no way of expressing herself creatively. Previously she had done a lot of painting but this had died on her. She was really just going through the motions of being alive.

Again we went up to the bedroom, and I started to use the system I had been taught. Energy follows thought, so I had to choose the correct colours mentally and direct them to the patient by thought, letting the energy flow through my hands. As this lass was so depressed, her entire energy pattern was dimmed and clouded. So it seemed appropriate to follow the full teaching schema I had been given, a charted picture of specific colours to specific areas.

When I put my hands on her head, however, the picture departed. All I could envisage was rose. And rose, in this healing practice, is the colour of love. Mildly surprised at using it for the head centres I nevertheless concentrated on the colour and pictured it flowing into her. Moving down to her brow, once again *not* the usual colour, just a strong affirmation of rose. The throat: rose again; the heart: rose; and when I got to the solar plexus, seat of emotions and identity, and still the rose persisted, I suddenly understood why.

I had no background knowledge of this girl, but I heard myself ask, "Have you been short of love in your life?" She started to cry. It seemed right just to continue, and for the next half hour, while she quietly sobbed, I flooded her with love: centres, spine, organs, nerves, tissues. Just love, in quantity, and in intensity of quality. I left her to rest while I washed my hands. As I came back she sat up, all cried up, but behind the swollen eyes she looked lovely

— peaceful, quiet, almost radiant. "Oh *thank* you," she said. We had no discussion — it would have been super-fluous, I felt — and off she went.

About three months later I had a letter: "Just to tell you how my life has changed. I am painting again, and so many things are happening for me. It's like being let out of prison and I can't thank you enough." Poor lass, life-crippled because of lack of love. I felt glad, of course, but also hugely sad as I thought of all the emotional cripples struggling stunted through life — when all they needed was the love flood!

The lesson she had given me was that it was increas-ingly safe to trust my intuition. I knew that the 'given' colour scheme worked well. One vastly experienced heal-er followed it implicitly, was never sidetracked by his intuition, and had no feedback through his hands. Yet his healing was powerful. For me it became a failsafe struc-ture (one does not live on a permanently tuned-in 'high') — but also a rule-book I could sometimes ignore, a bit like the grammar of the situation. Now I could begin to write creatively on my own. And did so.

This was the time for the practice to grow and take pri-ority. So far I had not advertised; it was all by word of mouth. But when radionics patients reached the fifty mark I had to face another decision. Was there yet again to be a leap in the dark? Should I let the guest house go and trust that one or other healing method would main-tain me? I leaped. The guest living room became a study and counselling room.

As I dared to make this shift, more insights appeared. One of my radionics colleagues became seriously ill. Intense pelvic pain landed her in hospital, but relief did not immediately follow. Completely wiped out, she spent most of her day in tears. Her husband, also a practitioner, rang to say, "Dorothy, *please* can you help?"

This request pushed me, I think, into widening my

ideas about healing through combining radionics and other absent healing. I did what I could with radionics, but every evening, after guest dinner, I went up on the fell and, looking over Swaledale, I just merged with the good earth energies, brought my friend to mind, and shared with her whatever healing depths I could reach. Eventually she recovered but I was amazed when she said, "The most comforting thing happened at night times, when I was aware that you were there, sitting in the chair by my bed." Was it true? *Did* my energy personify in that way for her? Why didn't *I* know about it?

The same woman helped me demystify more of the healing process. I had been told that for absent healing one should sit quietly, bring the person to mind, and *concentrate* on the healing process. This made sense, but not in this instance. She and I were away at a course for radionics tutors. Three of us were given hospitality by one of the senior tutors running the course. After a heavy day's work, when we were already tired, a hefty meal at about 8 pm finished us off. But mother, a dear old lady alone all day, then needed some light chat and entertainment. Painfully, we all trooped into the living room and politely attempted to oblige.

On this particular evening Sue looked dreadful. She had not been long out of hospital, and would have been better going straight to bed. "What's the matter?" I whispered. "*Dread*ful headache." "Don't worry, I'll take it off." Sitting at the opposite end of the room, I followed the usual pattern, going quiet and concentrating. My hands started to fizz, but I realised with horror that I was seen to be totally withdrawing from the happy socialising. "Get on with it," I muttered to the 'boys upstairs' (as we irreverently dubbed whatever higher energies might be available for channelling). And to my delight my hands kept fizzing, one to the other, as though they were still pictured one on either side of Sue's head with clear energy travelling between them. And they kept fizzing, while I joined in the idle chat, not concentrating on the healing at all. Better, Sue's face gradually smoothed out as the pain very evidently diminished.

This discovery opened up for me a whole new area in the field of radionics. One could give instructions, with intuitive direction, precision and clarity, and then just leave the process to happen. The new knowledge proved useful on many occasions. We had quite a long routine for helping someone about to sit exams — clearing muddled thoughts, boosting energy to the brain, giving relaxation at night, and so on. Previously this had meant checking the person out several times a day, and was therefore very tying. Now I could just write the instructions down, with times, and the whole process regulated itself.

Similarly, we had a very good energy antidote to the side effects of babies' vaccinations. So now, if a mother rang and said, "Joanna's injection is at 2 pm Friday," I could immediately write down the treatment, length and time on the baby's case sheet, and it went through when required.

Although these examples relate specifically to radionics, there was in fact something much bigger going on. As I deepened my intuitive access and trusted the information I received, I was constantly learning not only new ways to use energy, but also different ways to access the deep areas with which my inner Self was totally familiar.

And always I followed the Arcane School directive — that you deepen your beliefs through experience. Test out as you go along.

It must have been around this time that I had to reconsider my previous beliefs about time and space. My logical left-brain mode of understanding finds it just about impossible to grasp the concept, from modern physics, that one can change the past. The present, or the future, yes. But the past? Later I was to test this one too.

But right now odd things were happening with time. A patient rang up one evening and asked me to treat her. "But don't do it tonight," she said. "Tomorrow morning will be quite soon enough." So I left it, though I did go into the study and put her file on the desk, so that I would not forget next morning.

Around lunch-time, next day, she rang back to say thank you. "But you shouldn't have bothered. I was quite prepared to wait." Then she told me, in some detail, what she had received the previous evening. And the details absolutely synchronised with the treatment not given till the following morning. How?

I should perhaps have said time and space. For I was to discover that this kind of energy work ignores both concepts as usually understood. A young couple who had received quite a lot of treatment from me over the years went to work in India with their three-year-old daughter. I heard from them that little Marie had picked up a dysentery infection. Though the symptoms had lessened, she remained ill, remedies didn't seem to work, and they were worried. Would I help?

I immediately put her on very specific radionic treatment and, of course, noted the date and time on her case sheet. Several weeks later I got a letter, thanking me and saying "On such and such a date she suddenly dried up and, thank goodness, it has not recurred." It was the date on the case sheet! The treatment had 'travelled' thousands of miles in no time whatsoever.

During these few years, in the early '80s, I continued to travel to London for personal therapy and sometimes also to other workshops. I loved the visualisation method and became interested in a book called *Getting Well Again*, which described how a medical couple in America used it to benefit terminal cancer cases.

I thought over my radionics patients with long-term problems, and invited some of them to a once-a-month

Saturday group — a whole day to work with relaxation, visualisation and, perhaps most important, each other. As the group became knowledgeable about the method, and about each other's problems, the comments they exchanged were quite as supportive as mine. They also became adept at spotting chickening-out ploys.

One man had suffered quite a severe stroke. He came to me for regular healing sessions and, with difficulty, became mobile again. But this to him had not been the major disadvantage. He was a keen church member and had been church warden, sometimes reading the lesson and so on. His speech now was slow and stumbling and he had had to resign from all these precious church activities. Not surprisingly, perhaps, he had taken it one step further and rarely went to church.

I remember we did a visualisation where it was suggested that an important journey would be started from outside one's own home. Two familiar routes would be blocked, in different ways, so a new route must be found. The group howled this man down when he reported that as he lived in a cul-de-sac there was only one way out; it just wasn't possible to make a new route. (What a wonderful description of his attitude as it was then!). They wouldn't let him stay 'stuck', and finished up in imagination digging him a path from the *back* of his house round, quietly, to the church. It was moving, and he was stirred. No amount of surface talking would have reached him in that way.

I tried workshops too. The first was held one Saturday in the Methodist schoolroom and was entitled 'Healing with Colour'. It was almost entirely non-original, based on my own London learning experiences. It went well, and I was asked for more. So the next one included visualisation and a lot of additional 'openers' — drawing, role-playing, creative listening . . . Looking back now, I see that these first workshops were very much about method of one sort or another. I drew up very tight notes for myself, with detailed timing. By the end of the day most people were reeling. I did very little advertising, as many participants already knew me from radionics. Their friends came too.

Then invitations started coming in. One Spring I travelled the fifty or so miles to York to give a ten-week evening class. This one was the springboard for more courage and adventuring. Perhaps because of this freedom I was able to allow a more perceptive, interchanging relationship with those working with me. About time! I was horrified when, about six weeks into the course, one woman came to me in the coffee break, nearly in tears. "I *can't* visualise," she said.

How could I possibly have facilitated a course for six evenings and not seen this? Partly, I think, because I was confidently and efficiently dealing out teaching material (still a College of Education lecturer), and partly because until then I had not discovered that to share the inner journey means relationship, equal relationship.

The problem was not difficult to solve. "I always *think* the story," she complained. "Even the fill-in bits?" "Yes." "Right, so how come you choose those particular thoughts? That's fine, just a different way. After you've done the thinking bits, make up a picture for it — if you want to. Or notice the feelings, or the sounds. Whatever feels right for you *is* right for you." In no time, she was visualising. And I learned to be more observant, to relate more actively with the students and also to ask them to share their difficulties.

At the end of one session I heard myself brightly suggesting, "Would you like me to give you each a personal symbol to take home to work with, and maybe talk about next time?" A delighted 'yes' left me with a hollow feeling: "What if I can't do it?" And again, the small inner voice reminded me, as with healing, "*You* don't do anything. Just allow."

So, with the whole group concentrating with me, I went to each person in turn and, with the motive "This is for the person's personal growth and spiritual perception" in my head, asked mentally for the appropriate symbol. And the picture immediately came. It didn't necessarily make any sense at all, to me. But it did to the recipient, quite uncannily.

Then my outer life changed again. At this time, about five years after the start of my conscious inner journey, I began to feel a huge yearning for the sea. Reeth was almost equidistant from either coast, and my roots in Scarborough seemed to be *shouting* for me to return to that area. I still don't quite understand why I had to pull up stakes and move. I was only away from Reeth for three years, and it was a difficult time in almost every area of my life — mental, emotional, physical and spiritual. Or so it seemed. Looking back, I find there was so much experience telescoped into that time that maybe the move originated as a kick up the backside from 'the boys upstairs'!

The Life Flow again carried me on. Robin Hood's Bay was the tiny village that drew me. And once I had made the decision, it happened fast. The 'For Sale' notice was up for only one day in Reeth. The buyers wanted to knock down the price, and I was quite clear that I was not interested. An hour later they rang back, willing to meet the full cost.

I had not found a cottage that suited me, though I had looked over many. Finally it seemed necessary to choose one, but when I asked the local builder to check it over he said, "Oh, you don't want that one, you want the one on the street above." "There isn't one for sale there." "There will be next week!" And there was.

The builder himself was a wonderful, wonderful man. He knew every cottage in the village intimately, and was a craftsman of the first order. It was a joy to stand with him in an empty, rather desolate room and wait, in silence, while he considered. You could almost hear his brain ticking over. I finished up with a delightful, if tiny, cottage, basically three rooms, one on top of another, plus a six-foot-square kitchen and an adequate bathroom. The top room was my study and from its dormer window I was level with the seagulls (their 'boots' trampled above me sometimes, like thunder) and could catch a glimpse of the sea.

Terry worked all hours. Sometimes he would phone in the late evening and say, "Dorothy, I've had an idea." Yet he always respected any of my suggestions as priority. I was away when he tackled the damp back wall, set into the bank. So he took photographs of the intricate piping system which successfully drained away all wet during my time there.

And where was I while all this was going on? Once again, a Quaker contact offered me a cottage, at nominal rent, over the winter. It was handy, just one street down from my cottage, and I installed the phone, ready to take the number up the hill with me when I moved.

It was a strange and varied three years. For the first time in my life, I met angels, introduced by my first tiny grandson, who died aged nine days. I had never really thought about angels. Maybe they were just a biblical relic, something left over from my childhood when I had seen them in a variety of holy pictures. But this, my first 'real' contact, was vivid then and twelve years later is still indelibly imprinted on my mind.

My daughter was in hospital some eighty miles away, and on this particular night I was out at a Nature Reserve meeting. Normally I came straight home but, as luck would have it, on this evening I stayed for coffee and chat. As I came in, the phone was ringing. One of my daughter's friends was calling to ask if I knew that the baby was desperately ill. I put the phone down and at once it rang again. "Have you heard . . . ?"

Quickly I rang the hospital. "I'm the Lewis baby's granny. What news?" Sister just said, "Wait a minute," and then a tearful Mary was on the line telling me that Luke was dangerously ill with a hospital infection. If he survived the next twenty-four hours . . .

"Shall I come?" "Oh yes." "I'll come now." It was near-ly midnight. I had no petrol. I rang the owner of the local garage who promised to meet me in a few minutes. A great flurry of arrangements — cat, dog, friends at the other end — and we were off.

And then it all began. It was a wonderful night. I had to drive over the moors under a clear sky and a myriad of stars. To my surprise, I found myself singing the love-ly Quaker hymn 'Dear Lord and Father of Mankind'. The words were right, and it felt like a celebration. It was an experience out of time too. I discovered later that my beat-up mini had averaged eighty miles per hour.

Suddenly, as I sang and speeded across the black moor-land, I was visited by an angel. Huge and magnificent, he filled the skyline on my right, wings outspread, light all around. It was awesome. Then, as my eyes travelled downwards I saw that he was hovering just above the earth, and at his feet was a tiny baby. And I knew that small Luke had died, and was going home. When I reached the hospital he had indeed just gone.

The ward Sister knew how to deal with death. They brought us huge mugs of tea, and after a little while she came in and simply said, "Come and see him." They had emptied a little treatment room, and there he lay, looking very fast asleep with blue eyelids resting on his so small cheeks. All three of us stood looking at him in stunned silence. Back came Sister. "Have you held him?" "No," said Mary. "Well, sit down and hold him, you need to say goodbye." And we all held him in turn. I was surprised to find his little body still fizzing with energy, and found myself gently rocking and patting him just as if he were still alive.

After a while Sister came back and asked Mary if she would like the rector to come. To my surprise she agreed. I prayed that he would not come in with dreadful religious platitudes. After the angel . . . But he did not. Jacket over his pyjamas, he came in quietly, looked at Mary nursing her dead baby, and said, "There is absolutely nothing I can say, but I would like to be with you, if I may." And I felt that *that* energy was somehow related to the angel. Some considerable time later he asked if she would like a prayer. It was a spontaneous prayer from heart and soul, and was a comfort.

Because of the necessary post-mortem the funeral was delayed. I had had to return to work meanwhile, and found myself actually not wanting to go back for the funeral. I was not at all ashamed of the inevitable tears that might fall, but just felt unable to stand the desperate hurt and misery that must, I thought, be present.

I might have known. This time there was a whole flight of little angels. The church was full. There were toddlers and babies among the congregation. And it was still a celebration. I shouldn't really have been surprised at anything that might happen. But I was. The service began with a hymn for Luke, 'All Things Bright and Beautiful'. I had thought my fairly nondescript voice would be choked with tears. But from somewhere came these amazing bell-like sounds, ringing out across the church. After the service, the other granny turned to me and said, "I wish I had a beautiful voice like yours." I could hardly say, "Well, I haven't, but . . ."

From that short nine-day life, I felt I had learned so much about death. Fancy dying, to be part of that celebration! And about love too. I had not known so many people cared about us. It was easy to spot the ones who also had experienced deep grief. They said very little, just

"I'm so sorry." The others, bless them, tried too hard. Another lesson. Dear Luke . . .

In those three eventful years I also shared a close relationship with a woman. She had been a client, and had offered her lovely old house, in remote countryside, for some of my workshops. We had got to know each other very well, and exchanged visits — sea to country, country to sea. As time went on it became apparent that she needed to explore her sexuality, and was very uncertain as to its focus. Eventually she decided that her primary relationships must be with women. Our close relationship therefore ended — it was too much for me, but perhaps not enough for her. But she taught me to appreciate the great differences between a man/woman relationship and one between people of the same sex. Although it was not for me, I was shown how very intimately one woman can understand another, and also, I think, the unlimited tenderness and intuitive interchange possible between two women.

For me, this was not an appropriate focus. But looking back, the experience came at a time of difficulty in many areas of my life. Jo was a huge support in many ways, as indeed I tried to be for her through this period of her self-discovery.

Chapter Four

Jo introduced me to a different method of visualisation for spiritual exploration. For each exploration, one person was traveller, the other was guide. We guided each other on many such trips, and I still read with interest a book of records that I kept at that time. Sometimes the journeys were very simple, almost boring. At other times they produced beautiful symbolism, and approached the numinous. In all cases, there were insights to be found. Occasionally we recorded them on tape, for we found that the way statements were made by the traveller was often hugely significant and needed to be remembered exactly.

The method is very simple, but the person acting as guide needs to be well centred and tuned in, in order to ask exactly the right questions at exactly the right time and, perhaps even more important, with the right spacing. It can be quite difficult to sit beside a client who is working silently away as they lie there, and know when a question will be a stimulus or just a bothersome intrusion.

One starts by suggesting a short relaxation method, then asking the other person to imagine standing outside their own front door. "Describe this out loud . . . Turn round now and with the door behind you, describe that view . . . Now from the first floor of the house . . . from the roof . . . and then up into the sky for an overview." The description is always spoken out loud, helped by questions such as "How does it feel? Are you hot or cold? What are you wearing on your feet? Are you on your own, or have you company? Who, or what? How old are you now?" And so on . . .

Next one goes right up into the sky, out of sight of the earth, and at this point I usually suggest that the client finds ways of making him/herself comfortable for an overnight stay. This can be amusing, as I remind them that in their imagination they can do anything. So sometimes a full bedroom suite goes up there. Many people snuggle into a cloud, pulling it over them like a duvet. Occasionally someone says, "I'm not going to miss anything. I'm not going to sleep."

Then I suggest that morning comes, and I ask people to describe it. As mentioned earlier, it is important to note the language used, as the words spoken from that state of enjoyable relaxation can give strong clues as to current difficulties or, by contrast, creative potential. One busy GP sat up at the end of the exercise and said, "How wonderful to do exactly what I like." Many people love the freedom, but there are those who are afraid of taking their feet off the ground; they are threatened by the unknown and can't bear the dark. If this fear of darkness comes up during the imagined night then a question such as, "Is the moon shining, are there stars?" is often enough reassurance — though one woman insisted on leaving her bedside lamp on!

Once morning has arrived, I suggest that they let a cloud gently bring them down until they can see the earth and, instead of landing, just travel around the planet describing what they see, until they find a place where they really want to land. This is usually an imaginary place, but it need not be.

Anything can happen on these journeys. Some people have highly coloured fantasy experiences, meeting angels or other beings, landing on mountain tops and vividly extending their perception of their own strengths or potential. Others chug along in very ordinary ways, but the information that comes through from the unconscious is nevertheless exactly what they need. Sometimes a tiny clear insight, previously unrecognised by the conscious mind, can change a person's whole attitude to life.

The trip sometimes comes to a natural end, but often

people are enjoying themselves so much that a quiet "We shall be finishing in five minutes, so if there is anything you need to discover, do it now" is necessary to bring it to a close. I also suggest that they come back very gently and open their eyes when they are ready. People usually lose all sense of time during these sessions and are amazed to find that they have been working for an hour or more. Jo and I discovered that if we had a particular problem we wanted to understand but had limited time, we could specify at the start, "This is going to take just ten minutes." At the end of this period our eyes would flip open, and usually we had made a necessary discovery during the process.

Beyond being a helpful and enjoyable personal experience for me, I found this method a wonderful 'opener' for clients coming to work with me for the two-day 'intensives' that I set up at this time. Most clients knew what life problems they wanted to work on, but some came simply for further exploration of their inner life.

They came into the village in the afternoon, and we had the first session in early evening. That, for me, was a listening session, and we usually made a rough list of areas to be covered during the two days. Next morning we began with one of these trips into the unconscious. I suggested, "We know what you consciously see as your problem. Now let's find out what your *un*conscious wants to look at." The conscious motive might be stated very clearly, or just left open for general discovery. In actuality, I found it made very little difference. I no longer believe in coincidence. Somewhere in our hidden energy connections, each person had been drawn to work with me at this time. The inner material was just waiting to be uncovered, perhaps in this particular way.

After this first trip, we had coffee and usually spent until lunchtime following up and unravelling people's experiences. In the afternoon I always gave participants the choice of being free for country wandering and continuing work in the evening, or carrying straight on through the day and having the evening free. I remember one keen walker who got up at 7 am, walked all day, and *started* the workday at 3.30 pm.

Whichever time the session, we followed up hints from the trip, using many different types of fantasy exercise. And the day ended with a half-hour healing session.

On the last morning, we first checked the original list. "Is there anything we've missed, that you'd like to look at now?" We looked also at the way all the work melded together, one insight affirming another. Although I felt taping was not practicable, I did make notes as we went along, with a copy for the client to take home.

But the opening trip usually remained completely clear, like a sort of waking dream, and the insights followed for many weeks to come. I found, wickedly, that while I was usually very tentative in helping clarification — "Could it be . . . ? Might it . . . ? Do you see any connection between . . . ?" — sometimes a blatant statement, in my understanding completely wrong, might bring not only an indignant "NO, that's not right" but also stimulate the waiting *helpful* insight.

On the whole, clients found ways perhaps to change direction, they often came to see things differently, and once, I remember, there was a dramatic prognostication. Jeanne came for an intensive at a time when her life was in upset and bewilderment. A relationship was breaking up, she herself was threatened with cancer, her mother was very ill. How could she cope? And what next?

These were the conscious queries. And it seemed that her unconscious could actually give her the answers, although at the time we did not fully interpret them. When she landed from her cloud, she found herself at the top of a mountain, where waiting to play with her was a harlequin. And the harlequin taught her to play and have fun.

After a while, she decided to come down the mountain to a village she could see in the distance. When she finally reached the village it seemed deserted. Then she heard music, and following the sound came to the market square. Everybody was there, and as she pushed forward she saw that in the centre of the square there was dancing.

It was not a dance that was familiar to her. The dancers formed a big circle, with everyone holding hands, and the music and the repetitive movements seemed to flow together, causing the circle to turn gently. It was quiet and it was beautiful, and after Jeanne had described it to me there was a long silence. Finally I asked, "Where are you? What are you doing now?" And the reply came, "I don't know why, but for some reason I'm in the middle of the circle." "Do you like being there?" "Oh YES."

When the trip was over and we talked about it, we felt that this had been a clear indication that she needed somehow, in spite of the current circumstances, to find ways to have fun and movement in her life. The symbolism of the square-rooted foundation of her human life containing the circle of wholeness, within which she was centred, left her with a positive feeling that somehow this must happen.

This was not, however, the end of the story. Later that summer she visited the spiritual community at Findhorn. While there she was amazed to discover sacred dance, exactly the same sort of circle dancing as she had experienced in her trip. It all came together with a wonderful synchronicity, a bit like the pregnant cow I described earlier. In quite a short time, Jeanne became a teacher of circle dancing and started leading workshops which provided wonderfully creative days of dance and allied activities, such as meditation, drawing, sharing gifts, and so on.

Much more mundane and very satisfactory, although completely contradictory, was the woman who came to see me because, consciously, she was having great difficulty in her relationship with her husband. This was, therefore, the problem on which she wished to focus. As usual, we worked on material arising from the initial trip. On the last morning we settled down to look at her original list and see what we still might need to consider. I looked at her wryly and commented, "The one thing we haven't discussed is your relationship with your husband. Would you like to work on that this morning?" "No," she replied, "I see now that it isn't relevant. It's my son who is the problem. Why did I never see that before?" Off she went, and I dared to hope that their marriage would reap the benefit.

Looking back, I realise that I was being taught so much in those three years. Luke's death brought me to the fringes of grief and deep love. The female relationship gave me a lasting understanding of the homosexual culture. And all the time, although hesitant, I was increasingly trusting my intuition, while my spiritual understanding was growing almost inexorably.

The next lesson was illness. A protesting gut changed gear and started to scream. Visits to a naturopath resulted in vast weight loss but not much else. Finally, and I now believe mistakenly, I ended up in the hands of a surgeon.

Back came the angel! I was admitted to a huge surgical ward, and fortunately was blessed with a bed in a quiet corner — not that a surgical ward ever really rests. I was in such severe pain that an operation offering hope of relief was to be welcomed rather than feared. Though it was to be a fairly major undertaking, I was not afraid.

On the morning of the operation I could not, of course, have anything to eat or drink. After wandering around for a while, I settled myself in bed to wait for the pre-med. And there was Luke's angel, settling himself neatly over the top of the ward. His head was at my end, and because of his size his feet just covered the ward entrance. In an extraordinary fashion that big 37-bed ward quietened. I could feel the angel's energy unfurled, like a carpet of peace, love and healing.

I was enjoying this when suddenly I became aware of little darting cherubs all around the angel. And I knew these were carrying the thoughts and prayers of the many people who were thinking of me and wishing me well. They were gone when I came back to the ward, but I was still aware of the energy. It must have been reinforcing the specific energies sent to me by my radionics practitioner, for my recovery was speedy and uneventful and each night I slept deeply and peacefully. I had a brief convalescence at a relative's house before returning home. Jo appeared frequently, and neighbours came in to see to the fire and do my shopping. I felt well cared for.

And now there were other energy connections to be recognised. A friend who had worked with me many times rang me late one Saturday night. "Would you be willing to see someone tomorrow? She's a dear friend of mine, in terrible trouble, and I just feel you could help. I can bring her."

Sundays were still a precious space for me, and my immediate reaction was, "Couldn't you come on Monday?" "No, she has to have made a firm decision by then." Reluctantly I agreed to be free in the early afternoon.

I opened the door to a very beautiful young woman, holding the hand of a tiny girl. My friend, accompanying her, suggested that she take Mari down to the beach so that we could talk in peace. "Give us an hour," I said, and they went off.

While we sat either side of the fire, mugs of tea in hand, I listened as Lisa told me her story. Certainly she was faced with a testing decision. She was pregnant. Her partner did not want another baby, but this was not the problem. It had just been discovered that she had fairly widespread incipient cancer of the cervix. It was possible that the hormones of the pregnancy would exacerbate the situation, and if the cancer proved invasive it might be too late to operate after the baby was born.

She therefore had to make a choice between the 'safe' solution of an abortion, or the unknown result and possible life risk of letting the pregnancy come to term. The decision had to be made by the following day, the last permitted abortion date.

For about half an hour she talked and considered, and circled round and round the situation. What would little 17-month Mari do without a mother? Would the adult relationship break if she did not abort? Was the risk to her life a significant one? Could she trust blindly that all would be well?

All I could do was sit there and love her, and listen supportively while she talked it through.

Suddenly, cutting right across the dialogue, I heard myself almost shout, "What do you think of abortion?" One word came snapping back: "MURDER."

Silently, we looked at each other. "All right," I said. "Go and find the others on the beach. I'm sure you will find the right answer, and whatever it is, you have my support and care." With tears running down her face, she gave me a hug and was gone.

I heard nothing more until, late the next summer, there was a knock at my door. There was Lisa holding a sturdy baby boy. I opened my arms to him and carried him into the house. Once again, we sat either side of the fireplace, and Robbie sat snuggled comfortably on my lap, wide awake but not moving a muscle.

It was such a happy ending. The cancer had not spread, and had been dealt with easily in a very minor operation. Lisa's partner had found the baby boy almost a magic gift, and all was very well.

Suddenly Lisa said, "This is quite extraordinary." "What's that?" "Well, no way will Robbie go anywhere near a stranger. And he won't sit still for two minutes at a time." We looked at this gorgeous small boy, and I said, "I think he knows me."

And I really feel he did. I find that whenever I meet any of the children I have treated with radionics or other healing they appear completely at ease and familiar with me, often to the great surprise of their parents. Wee Jamie was another one. He was born prematurely, and his father rang to tell me, in some desperation. They had had great problems in achieving and carrying through a successful pregnancy. Now they were told the baby had only a fifty-fifty chance of survival. "Can you help us? You haven't any hair to use, I'll get it tomorrow." "Don't worry," I said and went up to the study to do the work.

Before I got out the radionics books I just sat down and focused on this small, new, much-wanted bit of humanity, and asked, very simply, for healing to be channelled to him. Immediately, energy started to fizz through my hands, even through my arms up to the elbows. It felt as though Jamie was saying, "Yes, I need healing, I'm waiting for it. I want it. I'm going to stay." I had never before felt healing almost being grabbed, with need, and I sat for some time, experiencing the flow, before turning to the radionic rates needed to help his heart, lungs and circulation.

Next morning the phone rang again to say that Jamie's mother had been woken early by the night staff asking if she would like to come and hold the baby for a few minutes. His heart had steadied, his breathing improved, and it was safe to have quick contact outside the incubator.

I was not really surprised. The connection had been enormous. But he was not out of the wood yet. We battled with infections, even meningitis, but he sailed through and today is a normal cheeky little boy.

When he was a few months old, his parents brought him to see me. It was a very hot day, so we stripped him off and laid him on a rug in the garden, shaded by a large umbrella. He kicked and gurgled, a small baby but very firm and solid. After we had had our cup of tea his mother gave him a little suck, then handed him over to me. And again, as with Robbie, he settled down, wide awake and peacefully still. And again his mother said in surprise, "He's usually very cranky at this time of day. I've never seen him so settled." After that deep, non-verbal communication on the first day of his life, I was not surprised!

And it is not just babies. A five-year-old girl with a serious chronic disability was treated by me for some years. She was a sensitive child and could actually intuit the colours I was sending her. We only met once, but she still writes and sends me funny little presents.

Animals also recognise this healing relationship. My new neighbours had two cats, a stripey one called Tiger and a ginger TC (top cat). TC, I was told, would have nothing to do with strangers, and shrank even from known relations. One morning they came downstairs to find him stretched out on the sofa, refusing to move. Something was wrong, and they hurried him off to the vet. At the same time, I gave him healing. He recovered fairly quickly, and a couple of days later I popped in next door to see how he was getting on. A small ginger head looked round the door and then, to the open-mouthed astonishment of his owners, TC stalked across the room and, purring, rubbed himself round my legs. He knew.

So why, oh why, do we as adult human beings try to break the flow of natural healing energy that *can* flow between us in support and caring?

Chapter Five

That same energy, if only we will accept and allow it, flows between all life. Some thirty miles from my present home there is an arboretum. Acres and acres of grounds belonging to a 'stately home' have been opened to the public. It is a quiet place to wander and feel peace and belonging. Thousands and thousands of trees grow there, and in the Spring every type of daffodil and narcissus flourishes between them. Blossom succeeds blossom, and drifts of bluebells flow between pink and white clad trees. In the lake are little islands, some with bridges. Nor is the individual forgotten. There is Jenny's walk, Catherine's walk, Henry's island. At one spot there is a whole collection of graves for well-loved dogs, resting where they so often must have walked. In the autumn the colours are beyond belief — carpets of fallen coloured leaves echo the flashes of yellow, red and orange shining down from the trees.

But the best part is perhaps the preserved wildness. The wide paths and occasional open spaces are just cut grass. In between the trees every kind of wild flower flourishes in season — celandines, wood anemones, primroses, daisies, an endless variety as the year goes on. Walking through the little entrance tea-room, ticket safely in hand, I am always surprised at the sudden recognition of peace, growth and sheer joy of life that hits me as I start my wandering. Often I take my cup of tea out and sit at the simple wooden table and just let the atmosphere soak into my being. The birdsong is amazing. What a safe place to sing! Later I may sit on one of the islands watching the reflections in the water, then move to another seat where I sit almost dazed by the scent of blossom. Or I watch a frog steadily jumping across a piece of lawn. At one stage in the Spring it is almost impossible to walk on some of the paths for mating frogs!

In this place it feels as if time has stopped, or maybe it is just 'out of time'. There can be many cars parked outside, but inside the paths are so many and various that only occasionally do you meet someone else wandering around. Nor is there any sense of hurry. People take the time to stop to look at an exceptional blossom or a lovely shape or colour. Inevitably there have to be the eager beavers armed with catalogues and needing factual knowledge, but even they walk slowly, quietly, gently, as they cover the ground.

I find myself talking to the trees. They are so beautiful, so alive, so apparently different from me in energy. And yet we belong to each other. One day I sat quietly on a seat opposite some huge blue cypresses. I was not very well and it struck me that it must be healing to exchange energy with these vast and wonderful examples of aliveness. So I imagined energy coming up from the roots of one of the trees, way down in the depths of the earth, travelling up its massive trunk and shooting up into the sky, then circling over and quietly entering my head, down through my body, and out into the earth through my feet, there to circle under and repeat the process. I sat for some time feeling this circular flow and then, looking at the top of the tree, was surprised to 'see' a great burst of gold and deep healing blue each time the energy shot up. In typical 'little me' fashion, I wanted to pin it down more. "What colour comes down into me?" The answer was a bit like a slap to a naughty child: "Watch the blue and gold, and never mind."

It is so easy to communicate in that place. A tree to hug, give energy, get energy. Perhaps the tree energy includes rooted stability? Perhaps my energy is to do with free movement? I can't know, but I am quite sure the enjoyment is mutual. I find a lovely flower to touch and love, or I offer a spoken thank you to a particularly beautiful blossom tree. And scent . . . I often think that the spirit of a flower is expressed in its scent. Some scents we are not sensitive enough to appreciate. But in lilac time, for example, the waves of scent from the pale lavender flowers seem to shout to my spirit. As I touch and smell them, we greet each other in a very special way.

This place is for me like a pocket of refuge in a busy, hurried, competitive, sometimes sick world. Every time I visit it, I think, "If *everyone* could truly experience this, there could never be war." And then I think, "Yes, and if we could really use this energy, consistently, in our private lives . . . ?" Never mind, it is a reminder that Life is, and its isness can be thus if we are not too obstructive.

Further threads of inner communication were about to become apparent as I hit a hard patch in the outer journey. After my long illness and convalescence, my finances were at rock bottom. Slowly I began to rebuild my inevitably diminished practice. Then one day a friend suggested, "Why don't you do readings?" I recoiled instantly. Readings, to me, were allied to teacups, fortune telling and ego-tripping psychic phenomena. I wanted none of it. But she persisted. "I don't mean *that* kind of reading. More to do with healing. You could use your visualisation skills as the method, and call on your intuition for the material. It would be more like a truncated one-to-one healing session."

The idea twinkled in my mind. Gradually it began to take more definite shape. Together we decided to call the first tapes 'Healing Commentaries'. Grudgingly, I stuttered my way through the first tape, which was for her, and then experimented with friends who I knew would be tolerant. Little did I realise that in the next twelve years I would record five hundred 'Personal Tapes' before finally closing the book on that particular venture.

Over the years the format changed and the motive became clearer. Gradually I evolved a statement for the beginning of each tape: "The motive of this tape is that it will help you in your personal growth and spiritual perception." And almost always this has been the case. Very, very often something somewhere in the content triggers a new spiritual insight, confirms a half-sensed aim or hope, or finally defeats a long-held doubt.

I say 'almost'. I remember with a sort of wry amusement the man who had been strongly advised by his therapist to send for one of my tapes. I cannot now remember his name, or the theme of his tape, but it was duly recorded and sent off. A week later I heard from the therapist who said, "I thought you'd like to know the result of your tape for A . . ." Apparently he had appeared for his next therapy session gingerly holding the tape and saying, "Take it back, I don't want it. She must be a witch, she knows too much about me." I didn't, of course, but had merely used the 'given' intuitive information as a means of stirring his journey into progress again. Apparently, this exactly fitted his therapy sessions. Now his therapist told me, "I sent him to you as he seemed impossibly 'stuck'. I hoped you could shift him!" Sadly, just then he was too afraid to trust and move on.

So what were the themes of these tapes? And how did I find the material? Let's start with the themes. The first side of the tape was intended to present to the recipients some aspect in their life that needed scrutiny, in spiritual terms. It might be something that needed to be discarded, or something not usually noted or even avoided. Occasionally this might only be relevant to one tiny bit of their life which nevertheless was holding up the works. Usually it was to indicate some focus that would be helpful, creative and spiritually releasing.

There were some interesting themes. Glancing through my brief notes, in book four of the records I see 'Creative acceptance' (the emphasis being on creative), 'Crossroads' (where do I go next?), 'Holder of dreams' — this to a lovely woman working as a therapist who, in a very feminine way, could be transforming her clients' negatives into hope and courage, holding dreams safe for them. 'Drop an octave' — this one was to a highly sensitive woman who did readings of a very different type, sometimes with an ominous lack of earthing. For a man, to look at his masculine femininity. For one woman, 'Tighten up'; for another, 'Stripping off' — all the years of clutter and a spiritual search so frantic that she was losing sight of the wood for the trees. A lovely one: 'Tend your fire' (which only needed a bit more air to blaze up and give warmth and light all around). 'Boundaries', 'Gaps', 'Unpacking' and the more obvious (though not to the person concerned) 'Serenity, courage, change', 'Living your balance', 'Standing straight', 'Allowing', and one for grief which I too found helpful: 'Sorrow is to hold — sorrow is not to be wasted'.

So the theme was laid down and elaborated, and then a short original guided fantasy was given, to be repeated many times for further clarification from the unconscious. Sometimes the theme hit a bullseye in relation to an actual outside circumstance, and this made even greater impact. One woman's theme was 'Pace setting'. Talking about it on the first side of the tape, I asked her to think of a car idling while waiting to move, then to consider the pace she needed to set for her*self* rather than for her job. Finally I suggested that she set an imaginary pacemaker in herself, to regulate her energy and bring her into balance. What I did not know was that she had recently visited her doctor because of bothersome symptoms caused by irregular heartbeat.

The supplementary fantasy was meant to help her experience different pacings. Coming from the unconscious I knew this would reach her at all levels. So after the initial relaxation I asked her to choose, in her imagination, transport for a journey. There was a reward for good timing in completing the journey efficiently. But then, with the same reward offered, she had to complete the journey on foot. What were her feelings?

The second phase was to undertake a journey where there was no actual need to arrive! No timing and no reward. What transport did she choose this time, and how did it feel?

The third phase was to imagine that she need not travel at all, but just stay quietly with herself and enjoy that experience.

Each time these fantasies are used, the resulting material may be different. For the unconscious throws up what is needed for today, and tomorrow's today may have different needs. Nevertheless, I wasn't totally surprised that some months later this client decided to leave her highly pressured job and work in a different setting. She got less money, but much more time for herself and her inner journey — and, of course, more space to let her heart-love flow without irregularity.

One of the more interesting discoveries in the feedback, for me, was how often we cannot recognise our own sticking points. It's as if the points are jammed, so to speak, and we are powerless. It just needs someone to throw the lever — in this case, send a tape — and the journey surges on.

Sometimes, of course, this means staying exactly where you are. A very much loved friend who has MS phoned and asked me for a tape. He has been wonderfully persistent in creative adaptation as his physical body gradually shuts down. But possibly at that particular time he was very aware of increasing limitation and frustration.

The theme I got for his tape was wonderful. I could *see* the images, and managed successfully to share them with him. The theme was twofold: 'Giant' and 'Authenticity'. I saw his spirit as strong, beautiful and burgeoning — totally fitting for a giant. And this giant was so authentic,

so real. Yes, life is difficult. Yes, life holds pain. Yes, sometimes one cannot cope. That *is* life. But if it is lived, not
shirked, not run away from, not abandoned, then reality
flourishes and an authentic life flows in, with creativity,
love, compassion and understanding. For all the difficult,
sad life-spaces hide gifts. I believe this, indeed know this
through my own experience.

His guided fantasy was very simple. He had worked
with me previously, so I knew he could easily find space
for it and let his mind flow free. First, in his imagination
he had to find a quiet place that was just right for him as
a giant — maybe a mountain as a chair, a hill as a foot-
stool — and there be still. Then he was to have three visitors. First, a child to give the giant a present; then a lover
to give the giant a present; and finally his own Higher Self
spirituality, perhaps seen as a Being, a person, a feeling
or a colour, to give the giant a present. Those presents had
to be scrutinised and accepted. That was all!

In this way he could see, first, that he needed to accept
himself as of real stature, a giant. Second, because in fantasy, as in a dream, all the different parts represent the
person, he had to discover what the child bit of him could
contribute to the giant he really is. And what the lover
part could give, and what he could receive from the spiritual aspect, which was totally in touch with the struggling and sometimes despairing man that he sometimes
was, although still a giant. That tape was a special one for
me.

So much for the themes. Now for the second question:
How do you find the material? How do you produce such
individually appropriate tapes? Inevitably, the short
answer must be that I don't know. There isn't a definite
procedure. I certainly never sit down and *think*, "What
does this person need? What ought I to say?"

It works like this. When I get a request for a tape, with
signature and date of birth, I just put it on one side and

wait. Very often it is when I am out with the dog, in the fields or on the moor, that suddenly the theme comes into my mind. "Oh yes, that's what is needed."

I let my mind roam freely around the theme, not thinking or planning, but allowing the idea to expand. The material for the accompanying fantasy usually comes at the same time, and I feel safer if I have a rough idea of the content before beginning to record — although there is always the pause button!

The second side of the tape is quite different. It is made up of a whole series of short visualisation exercises, ten or more. I suggest that clients choose one or two to work with, sit down, relax, and bring the chosen picture to mind. Usually I also suggest questions they can ask themselves about the scene, but I always emphasise that the picture is for them, not for me, so any connections they themselves make are right and need to be looked at.

Again, as in dreams, all the bits of the picture are the person. Sometimes I suggest watching the scene from a child's point of view, sometimes an adult's, often each in turn. Feelings discovered in this way — the hidden parts of a person's emotional life — can trigger enormously positive changes. For example, the vignette might be of a two- or three-year-old tucking into a huge piece of messy chocolate cake, totally enjoying it, with chocolate everywhere. The adult comes in. What is her reaction, and how do you, as toddler, feel about that? Second time round, you are the adult. How do you feel as you come in and find this dreadful mess? How do you react? How does it feel? And could this be a habitual feeling or reaction to 'mess' in life that is holding up the flexibility of the inner journey?

I was familiar, of course, with the different functions of right brain and left brain when dealing with concepts. The left brain works with reasoned precision — step by step by step, a living binary computer. This side of the brain is encouraged at school in academic pursuits, and is familiar to all of us — safe ground. The right side's functioning is quite different. It appears to see the whole picture (a living analogue computer?), and passes this on to us in tantalising glimpses and hints, relying heavily on intuition both for reception and interpretation. Worse, it usually presents its information in symbolic form.

This tape work really brought the difference home to me. At first, when an appropriate symbol came to mind, I would catch myself thinking, "You can't send that, it's ridiculous," or "What on earth can that mean?" or worse, "What good can a picture like that possibly do?" But in fact the criticisms were not valid. I remember in the early days when one symbol appeared as a plate of sausages and mash, my reaction was, "How can I send that to someone as a symbol to work on for personal growth?" However, I already knew that intuition demands trust. One cannot pin it down and know for sure. So I sent the tape, complete with sausages! And the feedback included the comment, "The symbol of school dinners brought so *much* to mind. Thank you." I found very often, in fact, that the symbols that appeared the most stupid were the ones that really triggered movement from habitual sticking points. I learned to tell my clients, on the tape, that while they were working with the visualisations they should send the left side of the brain 'out for a walk', and only let it back when they had finished. I told myself the same.

One symbol that seemed to me particularly silly was that of a teddy bear sitting on a bed. I thought (left-sidedly), "How clichéd and twee." I shouldn't have been surprised when the recipient rang me up to thank me for the tape and said, "There was one symbol . . ." It was the teddy bear, of course. "To me," she said, "a teddy bear is the symbol of love. My family broke up when I was six, and I went from pillar to post and never belonged anywhere. *Now* the teddy is for me, permanently on my bed, so I can actually accept that that's OK, I deserve it."

Months later this lass came to see me. She was tall, slim, elegant, and worked as a model. Would I have considered the symbol even sillier if I had known this? She got what she needed.

It was rare to meet the people who sent for tapes. though occasionally a client would decide to follow one up with a day's work. More often there would be a request for a second tape. I suggested six months as a suitable time lag, and some people continued for years, coming back for a third, fourth, fifth . . . tenth tape.

And what about interpretation? I told clients that sometimes they just had to wait for the meaning to become clear. It might pop up, all unexpected, when they were doing chores a few days later. Sometimes there might be synchronicity — as with my cow in the field — and outer events would confirm the inner ones. It was important, too, to realise that the symbols held energy of their own and once released from the unconscious would work for the recipient, understood or not. For they were all held under the motive that the tape content should be for the person's best good.

So this was yet another thread of communication. I became certain that, as I was asked for a tape, somehow a triangle of communication was set up. Our two unconscious areas of awareness met and focused together on the deep, spiritually renewing point of the triangle. It was from that meeting point that the material evolved.

Chapter Six

The sea was a wonderful stimulus at this time. My little cottage was well down in the bay. On a wild winter night you could actually feel the thud as the waves crashed against the sea wall. I loved going out when the wind made it almost impossible to stand up and the seagulls hung on the currents and then swooped away at impossible speeds. By contrast, walking on the beach totally alone as the moon made a glittering path across the water to my feet became quite a strange experience, very magic, almost awe-inspiring. I felt very, very small and insignificant, yet at the same time totally integrated with the elements, the birds, the crumbling cliffs and shining sea shells. It was possible to walk out to a far point of rock when the tide was down, and although still on dry land I felt as though I was standing in the sea.

The cormorants used to find a solitary rock, quite far out in the water, and stand like miniature crosses, holding out their wings to dry. When later they were ready to fish and dived in, they seemed to be under for an impossibly long time, and surfaced way beyond their starting point. One evening when I was out walking along the beach, a baby seal came out of the sea and rested on the shore for a while. I didn't disturb him and he was soon ready to return to his fishing activities.

It was all so different from the familiar countryside. There I could talk to the beasts and feel their hot breath as they came to me. Or stay still as a robin approached, even tempt a chaffinch to my hand with a bit of cake or biscuit. And the trees and grass had a totally different feel from the water element of sea and sand and water-based creatures. It was harder to get physically so near. Communication was different, but not absent, or so it seemed to me. All the time I was learning more about life-companionship, individual *human* beings, with all *their* different attitudes, beliefs and lifestyles, while here there were other life forms which seemed sometimes to have different cultures to share, though springing from the same Life energy.

Inevitably I was drawn to other people who were consciously travelling the inner journey. First I found a yoga group, run by a deeply spiritual woman. She was very supportive, and though some of the group were much more flexible than I was she always reminded us not to strain or 'try', just to allow the movements to flow. The highlight of the evening for me was the closing meditation. She gathered us into a circle and for a few moments we shared a deep quiet, sometimes with one or two spoken thoughts for focus.

Through her I also discovered a meditation group. This was held once a week at the house of a local artist. I was a bit wary of the type of meditation used; it tended to follow a rather flowery, almost emotional route. And when the session ended the leader liked to go round the group asking eagerly, "What did you get?" I occasionally, and probably unfairly, felt there might be a little competition to see who could produce the most brightly coloured result! But that may well have been prejudice on my part. As we drank our tea and chomped on bickies afterwards, there was a very warm and united feeling flowing through the group. To me, this made the whole evening worthwhile. Who was I to lay down the 'how' of the procedure?

During my stay in Robin Hood's Bay, the artist moved to a bigger house, where she took lodgers. She then had space to create a really lovely meditation room — very simple, with pictures and candles and a quite deep and quiet welcoming energy.

Our yoga teacher was a member of this group, and I felt very deep respect for her. She rarely said much in the meeting, and any spoken philosophy that did emerge was beautifully simple. To me, her spirituality was notable, leaking out into all her life. She ran an antique shop in the town. Sometimes when I called in, she would take me up into the store room and give me some healing. Amid all the clutter and odd bits of furniture, she sat me on a high stool and stood behind me. I came out into the street again feeling stronger, lighter and full of the quality she had broadcast, which is hard to define — perhaps a quiet joy would be the nearest description. Every morning she was up at 5.30 am and went jogging on the beach. As she jogged, she dealt with absent healing. All her life seemed to be so together, strong, focused and giving.

On one notable evening we were all sitting in the meditation room waiting for her to arrive. She was unusually late and we wondered whether to start without her. Suddenly she panted up the stairs, looked into the room and said, "Dorothy, will you come?" and vanished again. Startled, I followed her downstairs and out the front door. "I was just getting here," she explained, "when I saw a cat torturing a mouse. I couldn't bear it, so I stopped the car and managed to frighten the cat away. I've put the mouse in the car, but I'm terrified of mice! Would you deal with it?"

We opened the car door and there was this little mouse, completely paralysed with fright, stretched out on the front seat. Only its eyes flickered as I gently picked it up, held it in my hands, and gave it some healing. It was so far gone that we decided the best thing to do was to wrap it up comfortably in a clean duster and leave it to die in peace.

Back to the meditation room, and the session began. One of the group had just returned from a week's meditation course and very much wanted to lead the group in a meditation she had experienced there. The group agreed, but I found the content so convoluted as to be distracting, and mentally withdrew, retreating into as deep a silence as I could manage.

To my surprise, all I could see were my own hands holding the little mouse. And shining onto the mouse was the most beautiful blue colour. It seemed that something must have been going on, and I stayed with this image until the group closed the meditation.

That evening it took quite a long time to get round the circle as everyone shared their inner discoveries. When it came to my turn I apologised for not really joining in and said, "Pass." Two seats further along was my yoga friend. "Well," she said, "it was most odd. I didn't follow the main meditation either. All I could see was Dorothy's hands holding the mouse, with a wonderful blue light shining down on it." "That's what I saw!" With one accord we dashed out of the room and down the stairs. When we opened the car door, the mouse had gone.

The experience itself was startling. I had never before seen that amazing blue light. Why was the initial healing supplemented in this way? I have increasingly felt, as my knowledge has grown, that meditation is based on intent . . . of going in, of searching for a deep place, of moving towards the centre of things. What one *does* or *feels* is irrelevant, and may be a distraction. I suspect that the group's combined intention, following our united hope of healing, was what brought communication, power and a lovely result. (What story did that mouse tell, when it eventually reached home safely that night?!)

I also went regularly to Quaker Meeting — another group of people who were, perhaps, searching. This I found more difficult. In the small, close-knit group personalities were more obtrusive, and rules and regulations, necessary for any small community, sometimes proved very irritating. One man stood up and spoke almost every Sunday. His initial theme was almost always well worth pondering. Unfortunately, he did not sit down once it was presented, but added a 15-minute exposition which killed it dead for me. However, he was speaking *his* truth, as the Quaker saying goes, and I learned to turn off and ponder, while he carefully rambled on.

Shortly after little Luke died, I ran a five-day course on healing in the Meeting House. Each day there was a different theme and the afternoons were always practical. One of the themes was death. Because Luke had died so recently I was able to share my experience — and the angels. This drew a wealth of experience from the other members of the group. One member was in a wheelchair and we learned from her that an accident can cause a very real bereavement — the loss of an active life — as can a broken relationship, which is sometimes even more poignant than a death, for the other person is still present but not attainable.

During the week the students learned some theory, a variety of methods and a great deal about sharing in love (which is really the ground rule of every form of healing). As the week went on, the group energy consolidated. We began to have enough trust really to be vulnerable and this affected the healing practice, which sometimes took place in twos or threes and at other times as an entire group. And of course increasingly I became a facilitator — sharing and encouraging — rather than a leader who instructed and expected to be followed.

One of the students lived in a vast old house high above the town and she gave board and lodging, camping fashion, to the others. We worked hard all morning, had a two-hour lunch break for sea, sands or a nap, and then worked for a further two or three hours in the afternoon. On the final day, we got together for a giant evening meal, relaxation and fun, with a great sense of appreciation for the unity we had developed as the days went by.

This had not been so in the beginning. On the first afternoon I had unthinkingly directed people to break up into pairs — going round the circle saying you and you, you and you, and so on. Next morning I was approached by two students who made a very strong plea not to have to work with so and so, and so and so. I realised with dismay that this was not so much a personality thing as a genuine clash of energies. With future groups I always explained this: "If you don't feel comfortable working with one person, say so. It doesn't mean you don't like them, or are rejecting them. Right now your two energies aren't compatible to flow together. You don't need to let it carry bad feeling." This was another lesson, in ordinary life relationships, for *me* to learn.

In spite of making friends, loving the sea and being near some of my family, gradually I realised that this time was over and I needed to return to Reeth. The house in Robin Hood's Bay sold quite quickly and for a remarkably good price. But the other end was a different story. I just could not find a suitable house.

A friend let me use her holiday cottage in Reeth over the winter. It had no central heating and the bath tended to freeze in the bathroom extension. But there was a coal fire, and I paid to change one ancient bedroom socket to three-pin, so that I could use a fan heater when necessary. It was a funny little cottage, interwoven with the main house. My front door was at the back, and because we were on a hill my living room at the front was on the first floor, over the main house kitchen. The rent was nominal, and I put in my own phone and settled down quite happily to wait for the right house to come up for sale.

The next phase in my outer life was horrific. Looking back, I am still not sure what lesson I was meant to learn, and whether I have learned it. A tiny barn in a mews just off the one main street was being converted to a house by a local builder. He had done many such conversions in the neighbourhood and I went to look at some of them, and liked them. The price he was asking for this one was within my means, though only just. Before I actually signed a contract I checked with some of the long-term locals to be sure that his work was reliable. I was assured that it was, so I went ahead.

The building was done in stages, each stage being passed by a building society surveyor for the next portion of mortgage payment. I paid initially for the actual barn and land. The builder had just shelled it all out, dug the main service trenches and put on the roof when he came to me to say he had bad news. He was going bankrupt.

What should I do? The completed shell might sell, and I would get my money back. But it might not, and I had nowhere else to go. The summer season would soon lose me my temporary cottage accommodation. And if another builder took over at this stage, the cost would be more than I could afford. The bankrupt builder said he could perhaps stay on, with two of his men, working as self-employed and duly finish it. This would mean I would have to draw cash each week to pay for wages and materials. It was hair-raising.

My solicitor confessed he had sleepless nights, not knowing what to advise. Finally I decided to go ahead again.

I have no way now of knowing whether or not this was the right decision. Costs mounted and mounted. One of the men told me that the builder was setting himself up in tools again, through my money. It turned out, too, that this was not the first time he had gone bankrupt. And he had hoodwinked the village and local area to the extent of many thousands of pounds. I had got off lightly.

Eventually, with the house nearly finished, I sacked him and moved in. There was still a lot to do. The plumbing was a jumble, the central heating non-existent, and there were all sorts of bits and pieces to sort out. My finance ran out and I was in despair.

The only solution seemed to be to sell, even at this

stage, take a big loss and move — *any*where I could find cheap housing. I wrote to tell my children and asked for help. They were not interested. I discovered later that my business tycoon son thought I deserved to be in a mess, indulging in stupid quackery instead of remaining in a safe, well-paid teaching job till retirement.

Out of all the misery and fear, this lack of response from my children was a huge grief. I could not believe it. I absolutely do not believe that one's children *owe* one anything. But I was startled at the absolutely total disregard of my brief letter telling them of my plight — too brief, I expect; I was too depressed at this stage to launch into long, detailed accounts. And on the phone I tended to burst into tears. It taught me two things: never expect anything, even from close relatives, and watch out that you yourself are not likewise neglectful of the needs of others. That stuck.

However, my friends, surprised at the lack of family support and determined not to let me be driven out of the village, got together and gave and lent with huge generosity. One of my brothers finally bailed me out, and by the end of the year the completed cottage was mine.

It was a lovely cottage. The builder had been a rogue manipulator, but his design was first class. The big living room used the whole of the little barn, and the kitchen and bathroom were tacked on in what had been stalls for the animals. Upstairs, I had a pleasant bedroom and a tiny study, complete with a 2'3" bed, made to double as a couch.

It felt good. I was the first person to live in this house and it soon became energised in a healing way. The great stone chimney breast rose from the hearth, with ledges climbing up one side for plants or ornaments and a plateau on the other side holding a small television. It felt like a strong symbol for the heart of the house.

At the back was a tiny stone-walled enclosure. A wonderful stonewaller came to mend the walls and his men dug over and manured the ground. Later we had fun with a clothes peg and rope to mark out the little circular lawn, another symbol quickly flourishing in turf.

The garden took shape very quickly. The kitchen door opened onto a little patio tucked in behind the stone-built boiler house/garden shed. All my friends gave me cuttings and every one grew. Two great rows of raspberries at the back made a shielding hedge, and I put in a little rowan tree — to keep off evil spirits, perhaps!

Finally settled, I found myself in a space that was totally compatible with my chosen work — which I then proceeded to extend by attending two short courses in hypnotism and hypnotherapy. At that time I had great doubts about the use of hypnotism, and was also afraid of having it practised on me. Nevertheless, it seemed to be something I needed to know more about. So I took the plunge.

I thoroughly enjoyed the two weeks' study. We worked very long hours and did masses of practical work. The courses were well organised. We were given folders at the start and then printouts with each lecture, so did not need to take any notes. The demonstrations were fascinating, and sometimes outside people were brought in, so that we could practise on them, and also to show that there was no pre-session preparation. One such case was a young man who had travelled from somewhere in the south of England to deliver an enormous television suitable for group video watching. During the lunch break our tutor had discovered that he travelled thousands of miles each week in this job, mainly on motorways. He regularly drove at around a hundred miles an hour, just to cover the necessary distances, and had become almost paralysed with fear at the constant danger to himself and others. In spite of negotiating for more reasonable journeys the fear remained, and he was seriously considering giving up his job.

This was a heaven-sent opportunity for demonstration, and certainly there had been no opportunity for pre-planning. We watched fascinated as first he was deeply hypnotised and then told to imagine his fear as a tiny man, small enough to sit on his hand. He was asked to move his hand around, while the man was on it, and it was evident that to him the situation was totally real. "Now," said the tutor, "your little man is going to behave like a clown, doing funny tricks, pulling ridiculous faces. Watch him and enjoy the fun. Laugh at him if you like." And soon the young man was smiling away, with the odd chuckle. "Right," said the tutor, "next time you begin to feel afraid, you will see your little clown, and it will all seem ridiculous."

He told us that once you can get someone laughing at their fear, it completely loses its power over them. He then brought the young man out of hypnosis and asked him how he felt? "Fine," and a smile crossed his face. "How do you feel about driving back?" "Should be a good journey. It's a nice afternoon." "Do you feel a bit scared?" "No, why should I?" He went happily away, his life changed by this apparently chance encounter. It seemed that hypnosis could be a valuable extra healing resource, although for myself I still had considerable reservations about what seemed to be power over other people.

Hypnotists always state that it is not possible to make anyone under hypnosis do anything against their moral code or true nature. Frankly, I do not believe this. And I find it distasteful, even with someone's permission, deliberately to manipulate them from an unconscious level. So why did I continue? I think it was a necessary experience in both the inner and outer healing journeys. When I came home I used it for so-called minor problems.

One girl really wanted to stop smoking. Her main smoking time was with a cup of coffee. Rather to our surprise, the three sessions that stopped her smoking also stopped the coffee drinking.

The most amusing problem that I helped with at this time was that of the girl whose life was a misery because she was terrified of ordinary garden worms. She knew why. As a child at boarding school she had been held by a group of older girls who had forcibly shoved worms down her back. Logic told her, as an adult, that worms were totally harmless, but her current phobia prevented her gardening just in case she met one!

We had been taught a very effective way of dealing with phobia cancellation, and we ran through this while she was hypnotised. I also gave her a slightly different procedure, for luck, and then sent her away, asking her to give me a ring to tell me how she'd got on. It was Easter weekend and I didn't hear from her and feared the exercise had been a failure.

A few days later she did ring and said, "I've been looking for bloody worms all week and couldn't find any until today when I turned up a couple. "What happened?" "You'll never believe this. I picked one up and held it." "What did it feel like?" "Well, I didn't like it, but I certainly wasn't afraid. Thank you."

So for a while I attracted these surface problems and enjoyed the often successful results. Use of this technique was also very helpful in my necessary financial recovery. A friend in Leeds offered to rent me a room in her house one day a fortnight at nominal rent, to use for my various healing activities. Advertised in a weekly paper and in a Healing Register, this proved a very successful venture.

It was a journey of about sixty miles. I set off early, stopping for breakfast at a Little Chef. Work started at 9 am and I had 50-minute sessions all day, stopping for a short picnic lunch break and continuing till 5 or 6 pm when I was provided with a substantial tea, all amazingly and generously covered by the rent money. After an hour's break, I had a two-hour evening group and usually arrived home around midnight.

This was a very different way of working. Usually the method was visualisation and healing, Time was of the essence and, of course, had to include the client's initial sharing. Sometimes I did use my recently acquired hypnotic skills.

One little boy, aged about eight, was brought to me because he was consistently bed-wetting. I think in this case I did learn more through hypnotism than through the initial listening. We did the usual diary record of wet nights and dry nights. Then, under hypnotism, he practised prolonged holding on, followed by a quick trip to eventual relief. The improvement was dramatic. All was well.

Then suddenly, after a totally dry week, he relapsed and was consistently sodden. Something was going on! In the third session I led him into a much deeper hypnotic state and asked, "Why are you wetting the bed?" Immediately, back came the answer, "To pay them out." When he came out of the hypnotic state, we talked about his home situation. I discovered that he felt his older sister was the family favourite who got all the treats and was never punished. He felt that he could never please anyone, however hard he tried, and was treated accordingly. Thus the bed-wetting and totally unconscious retaliation.

When I spoke to his mother I suggested he should continue coming so that he could work out the underlying problems. But she swept out, declaring that it was a waste of time and money, and she certainly hadn't any to waste on him. Poor little lad.

Seeing seven or eight clients in the day, plus the evening group and the travelling, was very hard work. It wasn't so bad in the summer but on some winter nights, crawling up the A1 in deep fog, I wondered why on earth I was doing it? Basically, I was continually learning, and that was the answer. At that particular time I was attracting a very wide variety of clients — smokers, cancer patients, folk with allergy problems, with emotional problems, and a very few who wanted to explore their inner journey more deeply.

The evening group was a tonic! Eight women, very definitely looking for further personal growth and spiritual perception. For three years we worked together and the group became a truly creative mutual support. When we began, I used to prepare two, three or four guided fantasies to follow and we shared the discovered content as we went along. But as time went on, and the women began to know each other at a very deep level and to trust completely the group insights and confidentiality, the exercises reduced in number — until finally only one or two were needed to trigger really creative and meaningful inner exploration for the rest of the evening.

One member of the group always managed to find a baby somewhere in her material, even when this seemed most unlikely. It became a group joke: "Where's the baby this time?" It was not a joke, though, and this particular woman asked if she could come to me for private sessions, slotted in between tea-time and the group. Initially we uncovered a huge amount of pain, and the poor lass appeared at the group totally cried up. She desperately wanted a baby, but felt that the physical difficulties preventing conception were insurmountable. I meditated about this and finally decided to attempt to take her through a 'past life experience' to see if this would uncover the reason for the blockage.

My feelings about past life experiences remain mixed. I am sceptical on the one hand, but acknowledge on the other that extraordinary 'coincidences' take place. It is another area about which I don't feel I need to know definite detail. What I do feel is that if the experience related by the client — whether from a past life or not — releases negative energy thereby allowing freedom to move forward, then it is useful.

The hope was justified. The baby was eliminated from the monthly fantasies, while the lass's girth steadily increased. Small Laura was a lovely baby, and will by now be a lively schoolgirl.

So hypnotism, while definitely not a method I enjoy using or even can wholeheartedly support in some instances, has nevertheless come up trumps. Of course, it is important to recognise that definitions of the term hypnotism allow very wide boundaries. Our lecturer on the course told us that we all use hypnotism every time we influence another person through their unconscious response to suggestion or manipulation. Certainly I find that there are ways to use the voice, for example to induce relaxation, that may well be considered hypnotic.

Later I went to a self-hypnotism course, and this offered many very useful ideas, including a powerful but enjoyable method of affirmation — so simple, so effective. After an initial relaxation, perhaps just three deep breaths, letting go of current emotional, physical and mental problems on each outbreath, all that is needed is to focus on the symbol that brings the required material to the unconscious; and keep focusing for a whole minute. Then count oneself back to normal consciousness — 1,2,3, emerging on 3 feeling relaxed, energised and confident. It works.

As preparation, I spent time with clients to help them find up to four needs they wished to affirm. It was important to express these as positives. For example, anyone who wanted to overcome fear must not say, "I am not afraid," as this would bring the fear to mind, but rather, "I am courageous," and so on. In a way, one is telling whopping falsehoods, but we are taught that the unconscious is a 'yes' person!

This is where so many resolutions or expressed needs go wrong in our lives, We give hopelessly confused signals. "I would like a new partner." "Yes," agrees the unconscious. But then, "I'm not really good enough to deserve this." "Yes." Again the agreement! Do you see? So once the positive statements had been worked out, I suggested that they be written down (at one point I had copies in each room, so I could not get out of using the process by default!) and read aloud before going into the relaxation. Thus the conscious brain was imprinted first and then, with the request that all four statements be recognised by the unconscious through the use of the symbol, the focusing started. The symbol itself was discovered very simply, just by relaxing and asking for it to come to mind in relation to the written statements. The relationship between the two did not have to be, and often was not, apparent.

The usual affirmation method of writing down positive statements over and over had never appealed to me. It was such a chore and I never kept it up for more than a day or two. This new method I enjoyed and found easy, and I later discovered that just bringing the symbol to mind activated the affirmation, without having always to follow the rest of the ritual.

My day at Leeds was a Tuesday, just once a fortnight. I suddenly realised that as early as the preceding Thursday I was beginning to anticipate and dread the 17-hour day. A small voice inside my head said, "Don't do it. Just work from home." In a remote Swaledale village? Panic at the thought of loss of income made me put that idea aside. But perhaps through my meditation sessions, or perhaps through recognition of the situation as a lesson in trust, I decided this *was* the right thing to do.

Chapter Seven

It proved so to be. The cottage and garden were ideal for small group sessions. Even better, the little Community Centre next door could be rented for groups of twenty or more at reasonable cost. I organised workshops, sent out mailshots to the ex-Leeds clients, and began in earnest to run the two-day intensive one-to-one work sessions.

And clients came. With workshops, intensives and a new burst of energy in the radionics practice, I was as busy again as I wanted to be. A programme I found recently reminds me that I was also being invited to lead workshops over quite a wide area of the North of England. At that time the themes were related to healing in a fairly general way. 'Introduction to Colour Healing' followed by 'The Healing Space', 'Natural Healing', 'Dowsing for Health' and so forth. From there the Creative Visualisation method suggested more focused themes: 'A Day of Renewal', 'Focus, Centring, Serenity', 'Healing for You, Healing for Me', 'Healing as Relationship', 'My Parent, My Child' . . . They averaged out as two single days and one weekend a month. Although they were tiring, I found the stimulation and sharing offered more than compensation. And, of course, there was the fee.

I have talked with many healers about fees, charges, *money*. The comment so often has been "But healing is a gift. How can you charge for healing?" Somewhere there is a weird thread of guilt about this. But why? Artists have a great gift, so do musicians, actors, skilled business-people. No one suggests they should not charge. Gradually I found the balance between meeting my needs and those of the client. Usually it worked well. When I offered reduced fees, for example to people who were unemployed, I found they were the ones who said, "Oh no, I've got a little saved, I'll use that." I actually found that quite a pressure because I wondered whether I could give them their money's worth.

What was happening to my personal inner journey at this time? I was trying to affirm in practice what I already knew in theory. Once we choose consciously to travel the inner journey, to learn and to grow, then there is no chance to change our mind. We just have to keep travelling. When I said to all the participants at the healing workshops, "Think about it. If you decide to be a healer, then inevitably your life will change," sometimes I continued, "It's a bit like the stages in labour. The baby is coming. You are opening up the passage. There is a sudden realisation of the inevitability of pain and hard work. You want to say, 'I'll opt out now.' But opting out isn't a choice."

Each stage of the inner journey was to me another birth, with all the labour and pain — and not always an instant knowledge of what had been born. I often only appreciated it some time later when, on stopping for breath, so to speak, I was able to notice progress and a changed outlook.

One venture that 'happened' at that time was just what I myself needed, and turned very much into a two-way communication. An invitation was sent out from Quaker headquarters to all Friends who were group facilitators in some area of their lives — not necessarily religious groups, perhaps social, political or in relation to leisure pursuits. Various centres were suggested where initial meetings might be held. The purpose, within this Quaker network, was twofold: first to see if there were ways in which we could support each other in the now; second, to discover new ways or extensions of facilitating, from a Quaker point of view.

I attended the York gathering, which was a wonderful mix of all ages and both sexes. It was fascinating just to listen to accounts of what was going on already, and the day was extremely well organised. We had big groups and little groups, used a variety of discovery methods, and finally came together for brainstorming. Two big sheets of paper were put up at the front. For the first we were asked to shout out spontaneously what we personally needed and would like to request in actuality. For the second, what could we offer, particularly to meet some of those needs?

I sat there hesitating, until a man called out, "I want to meet with a group that is discovering more about spirituality." And to my surprise, and certainly without thinking, I heard myself say, "I'll facilitate such a group." And so it happened.

After a lot of planning discussion, we decided to meet for one whole day every six weeks. And I committed myself, as facilitator, for one year. The theme was to be 'Finding that of God in me', for Quakers firmly believe that there is 'that of God in everyone'. We met at New Earswick, a modern Meeting House which held a palpable atmosphere of peace and creativity. Kitchen facilities were very adequate and we brought a shared lunch — wonderful salads, fruit, sometimes even exotic desserts. The first meeting was far too big — about 35 people turned up. But on hearing what the group was to be about, just the right number dropped out and we finished up with a steady attendance of 15 to 20.

Mostly I used visualisation exercises, but as the weeks went on we sometimes included drawing, colouring, drama, modelling, even circle dancing — whatever supplementary activities anyone could offer on the theme of the day. And of course there was constant sharing and discussion, especially during the breaks.

What were the themes? Well, the first had to be 'letting go'. I suggested that everyone had arrived with rucksacks on their backs, full of fixed ideas, life experiences, old beliefs and so on. And I asked them mentally to take these off and put them by the door. Then they would be free to allow themselves to participate fully in their discoveries, without comparison and with an open mind. At the end of the day the rucksacks would be there for them to put on again. Perhaps they would have to make room for new content and would possibly even have to throw something out in the process. That was up to them.

And the other themes: 'What do I want to become when I've let go?' 'Where *am* I going?' 'Who am I?' 'Why am I?' 'My self, My Self' 'Choices, crises, and conflicts'. The themes flowed naturally from those of previous weeks.

Each day we started with the same visualisation. Walking in quiet countryside on a late summer evening, as everything was beginning to bed down. Finding a grassy space in which to lie down and look up at the stars in an indigo sky. Then seeing the Star of one's Higher Self, and letting a stream of light from the Star make connection with one's Heart Centre — at first as an individual, then as a group, until triangles of light joined up and the central Higher Self energy circulated, heart to heart, within the group. After a minute or two, the process was quietly reversed, until there was just the grassy slope and the stars, and a peaceful walk back by the river, where cattle drowsed and a lamb occasionally called.

I found the energy produced through this visualisation — obviously a lot slower and more detailed in practice — set the tone of the whole day. We worked from heart to heart. It was safe to be vulnerable.

At the end of the year the group wanted to continue, but my commitment was over. This had been a freely given commitment, financially just covering my travelling expenses. But I had received a great deal more than money from my part in the sharing. Nevertheless, I knew I needed to step down. And, wonderfully, the group continued, with each person taking turns to facilitate. When I got trapped in Reeth with ME they brought the group to the Community Centre next to my cottage, and created a joyful day out in which I could share as much as I was able. We had coffee at ten, and worked till shared lunch. Then I retired to bed while the rest went out walking. We all met again for a 3.30 cup of tea, then worked till 6 or 6.30, rounding off the day with a pub meal. To me, this all seemed a practical demonstration of 'finding that of God in me'.

This was the only group I facilitated that was deliberately looking for the spiritual and even indicated as much in its title. But whatever any group's apparent need and label, it always seemed to me that the spiritual search was what it was about.

The Arcane School work continued. Every month my meditation report went in. Every year the material changed and developed. I did not always understand it at first, but as I went steadily on I usually realised during my work on the next stage that the previous one had been assimilated. I began to know in reality some aspect of soul and personality integration. And this, of course, underlined the dualities in my inner/outer life. Much later I was to learn more about synthesis, but at this stage I noted with real dismay the difference between the energies of my professional and private lives! Working with a client, the whole focus was on growth and spirituality. I must of necessity remain emotionally detached, in order to be helpful. The sympathy and intuitive understanding were, at least in part, heart induced.

But this seemed so often not to be the case in my relations with an awkward neighbour or an apparently uncaring offspring. Then the energies so easily swung to personality enhancement, detachment flew out of the window, and 'harmlessness' was a sort of pie-in-the-sky concept — far too elevated for me to adopt.

Obviously this was not always the case, and gradually I learned a new morality. Judgement and criticism of others became less and — hurray! — I even managed to begin to avoid making negative judgements of myself. This new morality was hugely simple. It rested entirely on the principle of love. To be truly loving came first; action followed. It cast a new light on relationships, and the hardest bit was to learn at last to love myself and not feel guilty about it. Black and white rules bent and merged and the painful dualities *some*times approached synthesis.

The other learning at that time was that I actually choose my life. Could I really believe that — all the difficulties, pain, grief, as well as the joys and delights? I discovered that recognising this at the time of the particular event was often difficult or impossible. Looking back, however, it really seemed that I had indeed put myself into each learning situation. And — horrors! — if I didn't learn, it came round again, often in such subtle disguise that I was in danger of not spotting it till too late.

This particular lesson was clarified by the 'evening review'. It was suggested that at the end of the day one should briefly review the whole spread of the day's events, travelling backwards from evening to morning. No judgements, no fussy detail, just watching what was happening and learning the karmic law of cause and effect. Sometimes the review was done with a particular theme in mind. How much did I use detachment, or experience harmlessness or joy? Where was my service available? And, oh dear, if I had got out of bed on the wrong side in the morning, by the time I finished the review I had seen how the reverberations had possibly darkened the whole day.

It proved a complete and sometimes comforting circuit — I started the day with a meditation and perhaps also a 'statement of intent', and the review returned me to that point and released me for a quiet sleep.

It became evident that my spiritual service at this time

was to take the form of both healing and teaching. Already I had produced quite a clutch of tapes — part talk, part experiential exercise through visualisation. These were not personally oriented 'readings', but for general use. Each set carried a specific theme: 'Letting Go', 'Becoming', 'The Healing Space'; a set about grief, a short one on meditation, a shorter one on affirmation. Oh, and one specialised one was to be recorded later for people suffering from ME. As a follow-up to the workshops I had also produced a little booklet on 'Healing with Colour', supplemented by three tapes explaining method and theory, and of course including relevant visualisations.

But apparently it was the right time to go further than this. Many clients had asked for work to do on their own, particularly if for one reason and another they were unable to attend courses. This suggested a new venture, a sort of combined distance and yet one-to-one approach. Once again, ideas quickly came to mind, to be given form.

The work was presented as a six-month correspondence course. Each month I sent out a booklet and accompanying tape. The content was stimulated by my own learning through the Arcane School, but included much original work gathered from my experience as I travelled. In Infant School teacher fashion, I set it out in very practical terms suggesting records to be kept, materials to gather — paper, crayons, file, etc. The first booklet was almost entirely introductory, suggesting a weekly programme and concluding with an outline of meditation for the month. The morning meditation and the evening review were included as a necessary part of the course, and the first tape offered mainly pre-meditation relaxation methods.

In the following months, the material was affirmed on the first side of each tape. The second side was a complete guided fantasy complementing the month's work. Gradually, over the six months, the content deepened, with work on soul/personality integration, on learning to love oneself and let that love flow, on the beginnings of synthesis and our place in the universe, on concentration on seed thoughts in meditation that gave helpful focus both in and out of meditation times. On the sixth month the tape was a full hour. The seed thought on the first side was 'The heart as a radiating centre of love, and the radiance showing itself as joy.' Square breathing extended this thought: 'I gather what I need, to help all life forms. I breathe out love on all life forms.' The second side was intended as pure nourishment — a fantasy giving hints as to the next step, and then two fantasies to share healing.

This course was well taken up, and it had come at just the right time, for two months after its completion I became ill. In the summer I had had a violent gastric attack. Now I went down with a 'flu-like virus and somehow couldn't recover my strength. Finally, I went back to my GP who said, "I'm sorry, but I think you have got ME."

The grand name for this illness is Myalgic Encephalomyelitis. It is a devastating non-dramatic STOP. The symptoms are many and various, but perhaps the most difficult is the enormous exhaustion which is almost like fainting without losing consciousness.

I struggled on till the summer and then decided to take three months off — no radionics, no visiting clients, no workshops, no personal tapes. The six-month course continued to be sent out, and I also met demands for the 'general' tapes. Most of the time I lay around in the garden. On good days I took the dog for mini-walks. Sometimes I could only walk with a stick. Sometimes my hands could not hold a cup of tea — too heavy. I no longer believed in coincidence, so it was not too surprising when a woman knocked on my door to say she'd heard I wanted a cleaner. I welcomed her delightedly, and only heard later that she had made a mistake. I was not the person she had been sent to! Feeling guilty at sitting around while she cleaned, I started to polish the silver, and stopped. I didn't have enough muscle power to rub!

I think ME is almost always an illness that one just has to live through; nothing really seems to shift it. One of its huge snags is that it doesn't show. Many ME patients look radiantly well, sitting around all day. It was hard to face the disbelieving looks when, for example, I had to refuse to help friends with some project or other. I knew they thought I was skiving, and like all other ME patients I lost several old friends. No matter, I made several new ones among people who could accept the situation.

Lying in the garden I had plenty of time to think. I learned a great deal about perception. The flowers were an enormous comfort and the little circular lawn a symbol of the wholeness that I seemed temporarily to have lost. My respect for *all* life forms increased. What would it be like to have the travel pattern of a tiny fly that never could go from A to B without zigzagging to C, D and E on the way? Or to be a flower having to stand still and endure when invaded by predators and eaten away leaf by leaf?

The seasons made a greater impression on me too. The little lilac bush wafted scent over the garden in the late Spring, then relapsed to 'just green'. By then the lavender was out, and the sweet peas were beginning to scramble up the wall. I never felt a prisoner in the garden, and rainy days were a necessary evil in these months of captivity.

I learned a little, too, about crippling diseases. I could not knit, but found I could do tapestry work if I chose a soft, wide-holed canvas. This was a real refuge, as I produced a vivid phoenix rising, and a pair of long, thin pictures just tumbling with flowers.

With ME one's sleep pattern gets hopelessly disturbed. Because the exhaustion is so intense, one inevitably naps throughout the day. Then sleep is evasive at night. The library kept me going for some of these nights, and I spent

some time plotting a future book and many hours sending out absent healing.

My real salvation was aromatherapy. I was fortunate
in being able, usually, to drive the ten miles to Richmond,
and once a week I had the soothing reassurance of warm
oils, comfort and healing. During some sessions I just lay
crying helplessly, but the relief afterwards was enormous.
Certainly this healing lass kept the muscular pain well
under control, and I was very grateful.

Gradually I made a partial recovery, enough to allow
me to have clients again, though at first for one day instead
of two, and to continue with radionics patients. I learned
to balance activity with rest and managed to walk the dog
again. It is a very difficult and sneaky illness to balance.
If you do too much, the effect may not catch up with you
for a couple of days, just when you think you have got
away with it.

Inevitably, I then got patients with ME. It was interesting that they were almost always high fliers with pun-
ishing lifestyles. One woman I shall always remember
came from the south of England to book in for a two-day
intensive. She told me on the phone about her job as a
high-powered executive. She was still quite young, in her
early thirties, and worked hard every day, brought work
home, and often worked into the night. At the weekend
she had a really high social life.

The crunch had come when she had been offered a new
job, much better money, more responsibility, but more
time-consuming, to start early in the New Year. So when
she rang me in October, she said, "I have to be better for
February." She was intelligent. She had read up on ME
and knew the probabilities — but not in her own case.

Her unconscious knew differently. We did a visualisation exercise about 'Strengths', a rather fanciful but potent
imaging, which led her finally to sit quietly at the centre
of a 'fairy-ring', a symbol of her own deep centre. From

there she had to ask for symbols of her current strengths to come out of the surrounding wood — animals, people, colours, birds, whatever — and stand around her circle. Once they were all there, I suggested that they did a celebration dance (for being recognised), and then one of them had to be chosen, to come into the circle and be taken home to use NOW, while the others, recognised and therefore available at need, went quietly back into the wood.

When it was finished we began to explore the discoveries. I asked her to describe her 'strengths'. With an expression of distaste she said, "They were all little dwarfs, like the seven dwarfs, and they all had labels. They were sensible labels, things like courage, patience, trust . . . And I couldn't choose the one I wanted. He chose me, came dancing in and wouldn't go out." Intrigued, I hardly dared ask, "What did its label say?" She answered with deep disgust, "It said Weakness."

So her main strength for recovery was to allow herself to be weak! And because the directive had come from her unconscious in that dramatic way, she was able to accept it and dramatically change her lifestyle. She finished work at five every day, learned to delegate and never brought work home. At the weekend she spent one day resting, and had only one social outing. The new job was possible under the same plan, and interestingly she then found that life outside work had worth and moved to free consultancy, committing herself to only six months of the year. It was not completely plain sailing, but she did totally recover over the next couple of years.

Meanwhile I plodded on, with the huge lesson that I must trust the Life Flow and go with it. It was hard not to dwell on or regret the apparent loss of an active lifestyle, and even harder really to believe that the outer life was only a shell and it was the inner voyaging that mattered and would not suffer. I found meditation very difficult at this stage, so I trusted that as well and sat quietly in the countryside, opening up to Life in that way. Eventually, a friend and I started a small local meditation group which really brought me back into contact.

And of course there were times of despair and loneliness. I had no family within the distance I was able to drive, and lost touch with my two grandchildren. My daughter, though only forty miles away, was too busy to visit, and could not realise my isolation and loneliness. Within the village I had good friends, and the little Community Centre right next door allowed me to do a little fairly undemanding voluntary work.

I made some funny mistakes during this unpredictable illness. I heard of a weekend course in Newcastle on Spiritual Alchemy. A friend was also going and as I was being driven I thought it would be within my scope. It started on a Friday evening and I found to my horror I just could not endure sitting on a hard, non-supportive chair for the three hours. So, hugely embarrassed, I had to lie on the floor in front of the group for the last session. Next day, we took a comfortable garden chair and all was well. But as with all cases of ME that I have come across, I had to learn my limits and it seemed that 'stopping' and 'staying still' were major lessons.

I did also truly learn to change my priorities. I discovered, rather to my surprise, that my ideas of self-worth had always rested on 'usefulness'. And 'useful' meant 'doing'. Now I was, therefore, useless and of little worth, I felt. But out of the grief of necessarily giving up many worthwhile activities came the knowledge that 'useful' did *not* necessarily mean 'doing'. If the illness really did remain, or even in phases worsen, and if I was just going to have to stay in my cottage for the rest of my life, then there was still plenty for me to offer.

How? Two areas of activity came to mind. The first was still 'doing'. I had plenty of time — too much it sometimes seemed. So I could send out absent healing, I could pray,

I could write to people, I could phone up. And the energy of these often inner-motivated activities could carry great power. The second, which marched alongside the first, was to make my cottage a place of consistent love, welcome and support. I could be available. This was much more to do with being than with doing, and therefore more difficult. But when I began to get letters saying, "It is just so good to know that you are *there*," then I began to hope that I really was following out these new priorities. Could it be that they held greater usefulness in the great Life Plan of synthesis than my previous busyness?

Over the next two years I gradually regained my strength, perhaps to about 70% of what it had been. It was now that a phone call from the south of England asked if I would be willing to go and give healing to a young woman with lung cancer who lived only 15 miles away. I hesitated. Was I fit enough myself to take it on? The girl was very ill. I discovered that another healer was living in her area and suggested this as an alternative. But although they had heard of me through a very tenuous connection — Quaker circles — they were quite determined. *Please* would I go?

Finally I gave in, and so went through one of the most moving experiences of my life and learned again, very differently, about the death part of life.

The first time I visited Claire she was still at home, lying on the sofa. When I went to her she grabbed my hand, held it very tight, and said she was so glad I had come. Her husband, who said he knew nothing about healing, was there for my first visit. I asked him if he would like to stay with us for the session, and explained to him there and then that, as I understand it, healing relates to the whole person — body, mind and spirit, rather than just to the physical aspect. We cannot promise that symptoms will be relieved, but healing will almost certainly bring some change for the better *somewhere* in the recipient.

It was very simple, that first half-hour of healing. Just a quiet hands-on healing, first an aura sweep, then a steady progress down through all the centres. And a final balance. Claire was already on morphine and not in pain, but her breathing was fast and shallow. As the healing progressed, she became beautifully relaxed and the rhythm of breathing perceptibly slowed and deepened. This, I discovered later, was to be the usual pattern.

I loved this woman. She had a true depth of spirit and was loved in the neighbourhood as she went about her work as health visitor. She had planned many classes for the locals and was determined that illness was not going to cut short her creative way of life. There were no children of the marriage, and she and her husband were very close. He commuted daily some considerable distance to work. It was worth it. Their house was in quite deep country and when I visited, the doors and windows were open to garden and countryside, an ancient dog stretched out on the front path in the sun. It was very peaceful, very welcoming, and very hard to contemplate leaving.

And indeed, she was not prepared to do this. She made the very clear statement that she intended to live. On my second visit she was alone in the house. Her husband had prepared their evening meal, carefully following the cancer diet, left her a tiny lunch snack, and arranged for someone to look in on her. So we had a chance to talk. Initially, I thought she might get some relief from therapy. She talked very willingly. It appeared that her parents and husband had difficulties in relating, and she felt a bit like 'pig-in-the-middle'. "Sometimes," she said, "I feel as though they're all sitting on my chest. I love them all, but I can't breathe." What an unwitting description of her illness, which at first had been diagnosed as asthma. It was perhaps an 'irritation' that had turned into a much deeper wound as time went on.

However, having put me in the picture she decided

that at this stage of her illness she was too tired to do work on herself. I completely agreed. It felt like the old illustration of a glass full of dirty water. There are two ways to fill it with clean water — either tip out the dirty water (therapy) and refill, or just aim a hose of clean water at the glass leaving no option but that the dirt be flushed out (healing). So we decided: no work, just healing.

At first I went twice a week. The door was open and I just walked in to find her dressed and lying on the sofa in the living-room. Always I asked her, "Are you still determined to live?" Always the answer was a determined "YES." I felt it important to give her the chance to talk about dying, and I felt it equally important to support her in her choice to live.

She deteriorated quickly. Soon she was taken to the little cottage hospital each night, to have nursing care and oxygen to hand. But she spent her days still at home and our healing sessions increased to three a week. She taught me so much. The amazing sense of peace that came into the room as the healing session continued. The almost awesome courage shown as she repeatedly declared, "I am going to live."

It became too hard at home and she moved into the tiny hospital nearby. Her parents rented a holiday cottage in the area and spent much of the day with her while her husband, equally courageous, went off to work. In this way, desperately difficult though it must have been to leave her, he showed his support of her determination.

We found that the tiny improvement in her breathing during and after the healing session was a great help in her obtaining sleep. So my visits moved to early evening. Her parents went out for a meal as I came in.

By now the cancer had metastasised to liver and stomach and beyond. Her legs were hugely swollen and it seemed impossible sometimes for her to get comfortable. I came in one evening to find her perched on the edge of the bed in great discomfort and fighting for breath. I always quietly centred down and asked for help before each session. Perhaps this night my plea was a silent shout. For when I asked her, "Are you still choosing to live ," and as usual she replied, "Yes," I heard myself say, "I think you are too tired to *fight* for life any more. Life is an energy. It is in all of us and cannot be destroyed. It is a natural healing force, and all you need to do now is to *trust* Life, and go *with* it, wherever it takes you. Could you just allow, instead of fighting?"

We didn't have our usual chat. I just stood beside the bed and prayed that the energy I was channelling would really help her. To my great surprise, with every little puff of breath out came the word 'allow'. "You don't have to say it out loud." She smiled and continued. And I thought there was a minor miracle; her breath slowed enough to let her relax again, and I settled her into bed.

Two evenings later when I visited her, she was sitting up in a chair, easier sometimes and more supportive than being propped up in bed. Her parents left as I came, and she was obviously very upset. "What's the matter?" "It's Daddy. He says this must all be 'for my own best good'. What does he mean? And he wants to talk about dying. I don't want to. I'm choosing to live."

"All right, well I'm not going to talk about dying. Let's think about living. And again, to my surprise, as I looked at this poor, transparent, hugely brave and enduring woman, so obviously dying, I heard myself say, "Let's pull in some energy to help you. While I'm healing, could you follow a guided fantasy to do that?"

And so it began. It was a clichéd enough visualisation, it might seem, but that night it focused unimaginable power into that room. As my hands were near her and I could feel the energy fizzing through, I asked her to imagine a tree, a beautiful strong tree. After a minute I suggested, "Now go in and *be* the tree. Go right down into your roots, way, way down, and pull up the energy you need for your life from the earth on which you live." Pause. "Now go into the trunk, this strong supportive connection between low energies and higher energies."

At this point her hand came up and started drawing circles in the air — such weak but determined circles. "What are you doing?" "*You* know, the circles in a trunk show another year of life. I'm drawing life circles." Then we went on, up and up into the top branches. "Draw energy down from the sky now, into your branches, into your trunk. Join that energy with the energy from your roots." And again her hand went up, waving above her head as she sought these higher energies.

As we finished that exercise she told me that the tree had been a huge and beautiful oak tree. It was very evident that she had genuinely pulled in energy. Her face was relaxed and her breathing not quite so frenetic.

But I knew we hadn't finished. "I've got another one I'd like you to do. Can you?" And this one was all about allowing. I asked her to imagine herself as a little twig, and to allow herself just to be carried along in the river's flow, the Life flow. I gave her quite a space to do this and it was obvious that it was an unpleasant experience. "What's happening?" "It's horrible. I'm being knocked about, and sometimes I'm under the water and can hardly breathe." Her actual breathing began to speed up again and I said, "This is your imagination. You can choose what happens, in your imagination. Make a happy ending to the story."

I shall never forget how her expression changed. Accurately, and unknowingly, she described her own death. A sort of glow came to her face, that tired, pathetic little face, quite transformed now. "Oh, it's lovely." "What is it?" "I've come out of the river and I'm just lying in the meadow among the flowers."

I kissed her and gave her a gentle hug. "I'll be back on

Monday. Goodbye, my love." And off I went. But as I drove home I suddenly knew that she need stay no longer now. She had set the scene and could allow herself to go. My goodbye was exactly that.

She died quietly the following day. The prognosis had been that she would have to live two or three more weeks. I believe that in this case healing did relieve symptoms. It helped her to die. She was in the meadow.

Her husband rang to tell me, and to thank me because she had so much needed what I could share with her, and it had helped her. I told him how very much she had given me, and said I was so sorry that this time healing could not deal with the symptoms in the sense of letting her live. And this man, who had said he knew 'nothing about healing', startled me by answering, "Oh, healing isn't about symptoms, it's about knowledge."

Chapter Eight

After Claire had died I thought a lot about the duality of consciously being so determined to live against what she must have known were impossible odds, and all the while unconsciously preparing for death. I think the determination to live gave her strength to face this quite dreadful illness with enormous endurance. But this in no way interfered with her inner travels.

I found this concept, new to my thinking, of great comfort. Once we have chosen, consciously, to follow the inner path, then that is that. The journey, like the river, flows on. And whatever the surface turmoil or uncertainty or even disbelief, eventually this merges with and even enriches the inner flow. *That* is not spoiled or diverted.

I had never worked with a dying person before. I had never watched over and walked beside someone right to the death gate. In allowing me to accompany her, Claire had given me a gift of love and experience that I shall never forget, and I thank her.

In contrast to this enriching experience, other areas of my life were proving vastly difficult. People who decide to deepen their awareness, work with energies, extend their perception and understanding, do just that. They become more sensitive, more intuitively open, more soul-based. But the sensitivity that is needed in one aspect of life can be a real problem in another. And the understanding usually comes last. Long before, while still teaching, I had had a disastrous summer when a lithography workshop was set up at the bottom of our lane, and I became hopelessly sensitive to the vibration of the machinery. The two men who had set up the workshop were very concerned and used every possible form of insulation. Somehow this did not help. As they had taken out second mortgages to get the business going, they worked in shifts, so the 'noise' persisted day and night alike. I slept usually on my right side, and the hearing in my left ear, constantly exposed, was damaged at that time. In one of those weird coincidences, the year after we moved away the business folded and the noise stopped. Too late.

But now, perhaps because of the ME years, perhaps because of an all-round increased sensitivity, I was in trouble again. I became one of the huge group of people who react stressfully to an indefinable 'hum' in the air, from radar, from electricity, from telephone wires, from satellites. It is quite different from tinnitus, though often dismissed as such even by ENT consultants who ought to know better. Because the majority of people are not sensitive to these vibrations, you are judged to be gently barmy, neurotic or just plain fussy!

I found that weather made a huge difference. Foggy nights were almost intolerable — the sky became a sounding board. Clear frosty nights were almost the same. However, you learn to adjust and mentally turn off. Or at least I did until, quite suddenly, *every* low-frequency noise started to attack me, or so it seemed. If a freezer came on in a shop, my head would spin and then begin to hurt. Any generator noise, roadworks, even a tractor engine, and it was off again. At the final flare-up I found it a real problem even to drive my own car any distance. First my head ached, then my ears chimed in, and finally I became almost dizzy with the vibration.

Going on courses or on holiday became a complete gamble. If my room was near kitchen ventilators or a boiler system, sleep was impossible. During a stay at my brother's house I was at a loss to discover what could possibly be affecting me — until my sister-in-law pointed out that the very noisy kitchen freezer downstairs was actually against the same wall as was my head upstairs.

It took a huge mental effort to conquer the difficulties of this new sensitivity. Sometimes I almost felt panic in the night — I can't escape; how can I cope? And my ear learned to set up an accompanying song with tinnitus. I think I would gradually have adjusted but for the one insuperable problem. My cottage was in a little mews behind the village pubs. And one of the pubs, for some unknown reason, cooled its beer through a vast old-fashioned cooler, run by a noisy generator set in the pub back yard, only yards away from my bedroom window. As it was thermostatically controlled, it could come on at any time of day or night. Some nights in summer, because of the hot weather, it would stay on for hours. I would be up and walking by the river at five o'clock in the morning.

My cottage, with its little walled garden, seemed so perfect for me and my work. But stress and lack of sleep made me realise I would have to move again. I hoped to buy another cottage in a quieter corner of the village, but it was not to be. The house went up for sale precisely two weeks before the big slump in the housing market. It took four *years* to sell!

Strange, it was another lesson of endurance, an unnoted endurance as had been ME, because it was not recognised by anyone else. "What noise?" people would say. "I can't hear anything." It was some small comfort to join an organisation called The Hum and find I was not alone.

Somewhere, this sudden sensitivity must have been echoing a new and deeper awareness in the larger sense. Right then I did not find it, and my ear ached at the vibration of a tractor half a mile away, long before I could hear the engine in the normal manner. On holiday in the Lake District I remember feeling really terrified as I walked beside a waterfall one evening and the vibration seemed to shake my body mercilessly.

The great thing that happened just then was that I discovered homoeopathy as an unbelievably powerful resource for myself. Friends holidaying in the north called in to see me. Pete had been a GP who had added homoeopathy to his skills. When later he had been struck down with MS and had had to leave the practice, he had continued to work with homoeopathy. The day they called had been particularly bad, after a nearly sleepless night. My head was bursting and I felt totally depressed. To my dismay, while telling them about it I burst into tears. Quietly Peter said, "Dorothy, I can help you," and to his wife, "Take the children down by the river. Give us an hour."

For an hour he 'interviewed' me in homoeopathic terms. "Do you prefer hot or cold drinks? Are you afraid of thunder? Do you like company when you are ill, or do you prefer to be alone?" Bit by bit he built up the pattern of my particular energies at this time. As he suggested an appropriate remedy he told me that this was for 'me', not for my symptoms. In homoeopathic terms, this was a 'constitutional' rather than an 'acute'.

Homoeopathy is a total mystery to many people. How can six people with the same 'flu symptoms need six different remedies? How can a tiny tablet with almost no chemical content, but said to have high energy content, have any effect?

For me, it proves perfect. The right energy support at the appropriate time, dealing with emotional as well as physical energy, and sometimes closely allied to spirit, is a wonderful gift. But there is more. I believe, as with all complementary medicines — herbalism, radionics, reflexology, acupuncture — for real effectiveness the practitioner needs to go beyond the discovered 'pattern' and allow the magic of intuition to affect the final decision. Lily, the magnificent old lady who first taught me about healing, used to say, "I sometimes need to refer patients to other practitioners. And, of course, I choose skilled practitioners. But a good technician is not enough. I never refer them to anyone who has not got that 'extra magic'."

I am fortunate: my practitioner has that magic.

And it makes sense. That was another lesson. If one has a body increasingly sensitised to all kinds of energies, healing and otherwise, the last thing it needs is a megabomb of heavy chemicals. Sometimes perhaps drugs or surgery may be called for, but only in a whole context, and with respect for the entire being concerned.

So I staggered through the four years, waiting to move. Many clients visited me, and I recorded a great many of the five hundred personal tapes. Also, as I was travelling around less, it seemed a good idea to write a book that would travel for me.

Although visualisation techniques had been about for several years, helping people overcome cancer, HBP and other stress related-diseases, I had only found one book specifically using them to encourage personal growth and spiritual perception. This one was published in Canada and was not widely available. My own clients kept asking, "Have you any of the visualisations written down?" and "What can I read?"

It was time, in this period of consolidation and waiting, to get on with it. And it flowed. I had already tidied up about fifty visualisations in such a way that they could be taped, or read up, for individual use. All they needed was a constructive linkage and development. I was really astonished, once I got started, for the material seemed almost to be 'given', and the years of experience that I had behind me, working with clients, helped me clarify those sticking points that particularly needed exploring.

The title was not clear. I kept thinking of one, then another, and never felt satisfied. Suddenly I realised I shouldn't be *thinking*, I should be *listening*. As I sat beside the fire I closed my eyes and almost demanded from 'the boys upstairs', "Give me a title." Instantly it came. *I Close My Eyes and See*, and the subtitle was 'Vision on the Inner Journey'.

After that, I trusted as I wrote. The theme was of focus on the inner journey, and the material just fed in. In a way it was the gathering together of all the experiences I had been through as I had kept moving, sometimes doggedly. Beginnings, then letting go, then becoming — for what do I become, if I can once let go of my rubbish? What about the snags, emotional barriers and boulders? Who *am* I, me with a small m, Me with a big one? And what about healing, and joy, and thankfulness? In this linkage I again shared my own interpretation of much I had learned during my years of study with the Arcane School. Towards the end of the book the material became even more earthed, and I offered very practical suggestions for meditation, relaxation and affirmation. Then it seemed important to give readers the idea of sharing in their turn — in evening classes or groups — and I gave a few detailed workshop outlines.

And always questions, the kind of questions that can only be answered by oneself. How do I bring into my life the truly spiritual qualities — intuition, harmlessness, detachment? And how do I cope with discouragement, 'stops' on the journey, emotional pitfalls? What are my motives? What am I contributing to the planet as I travel?

If I trust, if I TRUST, then each day can offer a new 'now', a new beginning. And if we all connect — fellow travellers seen and unseen — then awareness *will* change, the planet *will* flourish, and the Love energy will take its rightful place in the scheme of things. I tried to present a guide to respect, care, choice, change.

I wrote every morning and the chapters sped on. It felt as though it had been waiting to be written. Typing took much longer, and the photocopying and the indexing . . . but completed it felt satisfying. Then came the publishing. I approached various publishers and it finally went off to two major ones, who kept it a very long time and sent very good crits but said they had 'no room now'. That seemed the right message somehow, and I just put it away rather than chase around any further. I felt it would be published when the right time came, but it was not then.

Suddenly, a firm offer was made for the house. It was lower than I had hoped, but I had absolutely no doubt that I needed to go. So much so that I completed the sale, stored my furniture, moved into a friend's holiday cottage at nominal rent and started house-hunting in deadly earnest. It didn't take me long to confirm my suspicion that once again I was going to have to leave Reeth, this time not by choice. I just could not afford any suitable local property. I had to cast my net wider.

I began to feel drawn to Teesdale, particularly the village of Eggleston. But again finance was insufficient, though prices in Teesdale tended to be lower than in Swaledale. I visited every village for miles, both sides of the river. The noise factor, of course, had to take priority and several 'suitable' cottages turned out to be near farm coolers or silage converters. One was particularly attractive and I felt delighted to have come across it. It was small, but the price was right, and there was a tiny garden out back. However, when I went into the garden I was immediately aware of an ominous 'hum'. I thought this must come from a large lorry repair garage sited some way away behind the cottage. I went up to ask how often the machinery was used. "Oh no, very little here; it'll be the Post Office cooler." Unbelievably, close up to the very garden wall was a small generator throbbing away to keep the milk cool in the little hut beside it. So that was that.

But it happened. A friend came to stay and said, "Let's go house-hunting." Off we went to Eggleston again. This time an old terrace house was advertised. Unfortunately it was not a day the estate agent's surveyor worked, so we could only peer through the very dirty windows. It was on the lower of two terraces, set high above the village, with wonderful views of Teesdale. The gardens also came down in terraces to the row of little garages on the small back lane. The garden for this house had been lovely, but was now hopelessly overgrown. The house inside looked almost derelict.

A neighbour came out to see what we were doing, and offered to let us look inside. It was dreadful. The back quarters were smelly and damp, the toilet was in an outhouse, and obviously masses of work needed doing. Which was a pity, as the main rooms were spacious, and the actual structure appeared sound.

My friend was full of enthusiasm. "This is what you need," she said. "It's just right — garden, view, no noise . . ." "NO," I said, "there is no way that I am going to tackle a renovation again. Look at the disaster last time." She looked at me almost pityingly. "You forget Nick. He'll see to it for you." I *had* forgotten Nick, her partner and an architect.

Bless him, he did see to it for me. He charged me nothing, drew up plans and schedules, consulted the local planning authority and, finally, organised and regularly supervised the small builder who lived just down the lane. He, in his turn, was amazing. He and his stepson moved in and worked all hours — from 8 am to 8 pm many days. The whole family was involved. The girlfriend cooked for them and promptly at 12 noon and again at 6 pm the two men downed tools, for only half an hour, and marched away down the lane for refreshment. But when I called in to the house one day, she was there too, wielding a paintbrush as they desperately tried to make the house habitable before I had to vacate my holiday cottage.

The end result was a really lovely house, at a price I could well afford, even allowing for contract gardeners to tackle the wilderness outside. It did seem like a miracle, and I knew I was meant to be there.

Another life change which seemed to have happened as necessity. I felt rather as though I had moved to alien country. I knew no one, and though Reeth was only twenty miles away it now seemed like a different civilisation. I was 'homesick'. Gradually I began to make a new life. And even added to my 'family'. A young couple living on the top terrace were ardent members of the Cat Protection League, and took me to visit a cat shelter. I made it quite clear that I was not going to have a cat! Inevitably, perhaps, I fell in love, and came away promising to return when I was settled, to pick up Harriet.

When my last dog, Toria, had died, I had declared, "No more dogs." But a few days later, when I visited the breeder, I found Lucy, born two days before Toria's death, waiting for me. Her eyes were not yet open, she fitted nicely on my hand, and we both knew we belonged to each other. Harriet was also waiting. Her mum, a very pregnant stray, had been seen by a householder but would not accept shelter. In the night there was very heavy rain and next morning the poor cat was found in the nest she had made of deep grass, now a puddle. She herself was lying in the puddle, with five soaked kittens on top of her. All survived, and when I went to the shelter two had already found homes. Another pair of chocolate box type sweeties sat at the front of the cage but I didn't feel drawn to them at all. Then quietly, from the back of the cage, a small furry ball appeared, her long, dark tortoise-shell coat acting as camouflage. She came straight to my hand and I had no choice at all. We belonged together too.

Now she is bigger than Lucy, and has a long-haired coat of glorious colour. An independent cat, often outdoors, she nevertheless has a purr like a lion and greets me each morning by rolling over to have her tummy tickled!

So I had a family. I also enjoyed the new Quaker Meeting, and had a succession of visitors through the summer. Nevertheless, I was lonely and still wondered, "Why here?"

One evening, as I sat in my rocking chair by the window I asked myself, "What would you *most* like just now?" And the answer was, "More family." My own family was scattered. I had a huge additional family of ex-clients who kept quite closely in touch. But I wanted a family *here* — little children to play with and cuddle. I wondered about putting an advert in the local paper: "Redundant granny is looking for a family." Would it work?

When the weekly paper was delivered next day, I was astonished. For there was an advert asking for volunteers to become surrogate parents or grannies, to work with families with short-term problems who needed just that 'family' kind of support. There was a phone number and I immediately rang.

It was extraordinary. It was so exactly what I was looking for. There was a seven-week training course, one day a week, and it was excellent. We had lectures from every sort of professional working with children. We watched relevant videos. We did role-playing. We discussed cases. And, most important, we opened up and shared our lives as we learned.

And I got a family. I played with the two pre-school children, took them out, or stayed in with them and let Mum get out. I listened and listened to anything she wanted to talk about, and was just an extra Gran. I loved that family, and I'm pretty sure they loved me too.

The second family I worked with was just like a huge present — a two-year-old girl and Mum, the size of a mansion, expecting twins. Then the delight of the twins. It was a lovely new experience, and our training group also met monthly as a support group, a treat for all of us, as by now we knew each other well.

This was such a good *ordinary* life experience — all the mess and bother of small children relating so openly among the turmoil. I was intrigued too to find that I could very easily quieten a small, cross twin just by the way I held him and *thought* him love. (I wish I'd known as much when my own children were small.)

But my first Christmas in the new house was abysmal. It seemed that all my older friends were away visiting their families. My nearest brother was busy entertaining forlorn 'old' people! The 'grandchildren' family was bursting at the seams. So I was alone.

Two days before Christmas I took myself off to my old haunts for the day. I treated myself to a Christmas lunch at a little cafe I had often used. The husband of the owner, still quite young , had died tragically two years before. Shortly afterwards I had been to the cafe for coffee and had happened to leave just as she did, dressed all in black and looking devastated. I knew from experience that often after a bereavement there is a queer kind of avoidance of the bereaved. No one quite knows what to say, so perhaps crosses the road to avoid an embarrassing situation. I stopped her and said "I'm so sorry. How are you really? What's happening with you?" And she stood on the street with my arm around her, letting the tears flow. Since then our relationship, though slight, has been special.

She came up to my table that Christmas, and I asked her how she was managing, and said how I hated Christmas (just then). She told me how she coped, but when she asked *me*, to my chagrin the tears slid silently down my face. Kindness got under my skin!

However, the lunch, though dripped on, was good, and I wandered into Woolworths to treat myself to a Christmas CD. There was a great stand of Christmas CDs and tapes — carols, jolly songs, party programmes, and also one different one. This was a boys' choir offering a very mixed programme. Scanning it closely I saw it included a favourite hymn, 'Be still in the Presence of the Lord', and bought it just for that track.

That morning, on waking, I had asked, fairly desper-

ately, for a miracle — anything to change the dismal
Christmas prospect. I suspect I hoped for a last-minute
invitation or something similar. What I didn't anticipate
was that it would come through a CD I had bought for
myself!

That evening I sat down to listen. The voices were wonderful, soaring effortlessly and seeming quite 'other'.
Then came the 'Be still' song. I enjoyed the first and second verses, but when the third verse came in, it seemed
as though the whole room changed. 'Be still, for the Power
of the Lord *is moving in this place.*' I could feel it. I sat crying, but not with misery, rather with a deep awareness
quite beyond words. I put the player onto repeat and just
let the music and the energy flow through me. It was an
affirmation of belonging, of synthesis, of inner reality. It
was the miracle.

Since then I have made a tape for myself, repeating and
repeating the hymn and then changing to the sound of
the sea. I am one drop. But I am also the ocean.

At the time I was convinced that this was the miracle.
Then I wondered. For in the January I met a man, a retired
teacher, who shared my love of music, my intellectual
ability and some of my interests — oh yes, and had a lovely dry sense of humour. Strangely, for impetuous me, I
was very cautious. We saw a great deal of each other,
though we lived uncomfortably far apart. As the relationship developed I started to think carefully. In my
mind, there was one massive obstacle. Julian had no
developed spiritual awareness. He called himself an
agnostic, was doubtful, even cynical, about energy work
— healing, for example — and was ignorant about every
aspect of the inner journey, which to me, of course, was
life itself.

Could I really allow this relationship to continue?
Could I be truly close to someone who did not share my
deepest interests at all? Was it 'right'? I had to judge 'right-

ness' on the basis of my own morality of Love and respect. I wasn't stupid enough to think that in my late sixties I would ever meet someone who had not got *some* strong life patterns quite different from my own. And this was the case with us. Julian was technological and his main hobby was video making, to an internationally respected standard. His small semi-detached house was full of cupboards from floor to ceiling, holding lots of 'things'. Much later I discovered this was an expression of his idea of security.

My house was a roomy converted cottage, spare in furniture, with white walls, an old brick fireplace and lots of space. Totally non-technological, it spoke to me and of me in an artistic blend of colour and texture. Instead of expensive ornaments there were crystals on the mantelpiece, and there were books everywhere. My one luxury had been a really good stereo system, budgeted for along with the house price. This truly proved to offer nourishment for my spirit.

Did these differences matter? In superficial ways they did, at first. Our first major difference was about the telly. He had an enormous 28" TV on a robot-like stand, holding a collection of video recorders that he felt he couldn't do without. I moved my little box on its dark oak stand, and we tried it. To me, it made a total mockery of the room, becoming the prime focus. I felt invaded, but tried to put up with it . . . 'give and take'. The other differences just came from two solitary older people trying to adjust.

I felt it was worth it. His great passion was his video-recording, and to me this seemed a really creative hobby which I totally respected. He very much wanted me to become involved, doing voice-overs and so forth. This appealed to me too, and I looked forward to learning more. And in spite of himself, *he* became intrigued with my attitude to life, found healing worked, was amazed when he could feel the prickle of energy from standing stones, transmitted through me, travelling up his arm. He commented plaintively one day, "You have shattered all my fixed beliefs."

I began to think, perhaps wishfully, that he was to be my good earthing whenever I took off on one of my 'spiritual' adventures, and that it would be all right and we would each give to the other. For all the time we had a huge tenderness between us, and an openness that neither of us had ever experienced before.

So I said yes, I would live with him. I wanted to sell both our houses and start again. He felt that the country here was so much my setting that it would be better if he put money into my house and we lived here together. We needed more room, so he proposed extending the unused attic and making it into his studio.

At this point, I naively threw away my caution. It did not cross my mind that anyone putting several thousand into a house would be less than committed. And, indeed, right then we did commit ourselves to a life partnership.

Settling down, I began to resume daily meditation, tape-making and study, and with that inner backing managed to see any difficulties between us as necessary adjustments. Change, to me, is always an adventure, often inescapable, but usually with a faint excitement of 'What's around the corner?'

But for Julian, bless him, change was frightening. As a very young man he had had a year or two of panic attacks. Since then he had determinedly held onto a quiet, safe lifestyle. But this was too much for him. The week before the final burning of boats, after a couple of months together, he blew — a major panic attack in bed that night. "I can't do it. I can't leave my own familiar house, friends, activities. I'm going home." I calmed him down and we spent most of the next day, both very upset, seeing what we might salvage.

But two days later, returning home to take various bits

and pieces, he created a solid barbed-wire fence around his safety there. He just filled his diary: evening classes, club, society, daytime activities, weekend bookings . . . all laid out. Stunned, I asked where our joint life came in? "Well, there's bound to be a weekend sometimes, or the odd Sunday." Emotionally reeling, I realised that my role was to be something like his 'bit-on-the-side'. I knew instantly that I couldn't do it, shouldn't do it, wouldn't do it. Quietly I told him to pack up, then and there, and leave. It was a dreadful way to find out that it wasn't a right relationship. And it was odd that I was completely clear about it, even though I couldn't bear it.

One life lesson led to another. We tend to believe that our souls need to gain experience through our ordinary human living. Mine must have been having a ball! For I was into an experience of grief quite beyond anything I had ever known. My head told me what had happened, but another part of me didn't believe it. Why wasn't his car there as I drove up? When I came in, why wasn't he upstairs? Half a double bed must be the loneliest place on earth. I got caught out sometimes with wild bursts of crying. I went to Meeting, but couldn't go in and sat on the seat outside till coffee time.

I found that living 'one day at a time' was no good — it was too long. So I divided the day into shorter periods, to coffee time, lunchtime, teatime, supper, bed and an endless night. It was interesting to discover who knew about grief and could be quietly supportive, and also those who obviously thought, "It was only a relationship, what's the fuss?" On a routine visit to my GP I was interested in *his* comment: "This sort of thing is worse than a death."

A month after it ended it was my birthday. Earlier in the summer I had given Julian a luxury two-day birthday visit to a guest house in the Lakes. It was way beyond my means, but so good that he had booked likewise for mine, and of course had had to cancel. I fled to friends for the actual birthday and stayed overnight. And had an amazing homecoming.

The women's group, understanding my pain but not knowing I was to be away, had visited the evening before. So on my step I found a bouquet of flowers, a birthday cake under a glass stand, presents and, tied to the doorknocker, a balloon floating up and declaring, "Age becomes you. You've never looked so good." Dripping with tears, I gathered everything up and went in.

Chapter Nine

What had all this to do with my inner journey? So much. It was necessary experience, not necessarily understood — even yet. But again I was able to accept that every problem brings with it a gift, and we pull in the problems to find the gifts. So what had the gifts been this time?

Strangely, I had sensed for some years that I would, at some time, find another close relationship. This was because I felt I had never as yet managed to be adequate and creative in such a situation. I needed another try! One of the greatest sources of this present grief was that this time I felt I had begun to learn so much, and lived it well. And it had gone. I wanted to go on learning. Nevertheless I *had* received a gift that had creatively changed me.

The second gift that I hoped would be mine eventually was the ability to deal with loss as part of a transition, as a continuum, as a death-to-birth experience. I re-read C S Lewis's *A Grief Observed*. The part that leapt out at me was the description of friends saying (as comfort?) "You *will* get over it." And then his realisation that 'to get over it' meant different things. If you have 'flu, indeed you will get over it and be yourself again. If you have a leg amputated, you will get over that too, BUT will have to make a new life as an amputee.

After Julian I think I felt like an amputee. I had chosen to allow myself to be open, to be vulnerable, to be committed — actually to give some of myself. That had gone, and I suspect that no one else can ever possess that particular bit of me. So the different me now had to learn to go on.

Out of this loss, the third gift was the understanding and compassion engendered through the experience of grief in all its stages. I went through fear, disbelief, despair

— it was just how the books described it, but now I knew it from the inside. After my daughter's first child, little Luke, died she wrote to me and said, "I never knew there were so many people in the club. Everyone seems to have lost a child." Looking back, I realise now that I could neither really enter the grief, or help her. I would do better now.

Perhaps a fourth lesson, or gift, was 'Life has to go on. Outside it is bleak and one step at a time. Inside, the river still flows and you will soon come to remember.' Rather stupidly I thought, "If I can just get through the winter . . ." It didn't work like that. As the days lengthened and I wrote in my five-year diary, I constantly ran up against 'last year at this time'. So in some life areas it remained 'one step at a time'.

For that Christmas we had booked a tiny cottage in Robin Hood's Bay, and I decided still to go there, even on my own. We had stayed there in the summer and it seemed a good way to lay ghosts. And it was. One hurdle over.

The New Year brought major changes. These came as quite firm inner directions. The first was that I was to close the radionics practice, and this was quite hard to do. Some long-term patients were my friends now, and I felt as though I was letting them down in some way. This was specially so for one woman about to go through the IVF experience. Over the years I had seen her through one successful pregnancy and three or four abortive efforts. This was to be the last attempt and I gave her the address of my practitioner, feeling quite guilty at my withdrawal of support. I spent several days going through and destroying files, and it became almost a symbolic ritual as I burned the little hair samples, 'witnesses', and sent the energy up.

The second directive was about the recording of personal tapes. For some time I had vaguely wondered if I should stop when I reached the five hundredth. It was no coincidence that this tape came up precisely at this time, and it was totally clear that I should stop. It was lovely that the five hundredth request came from a dear client who had been struck by a mystery illness and was confused, confounded and asking for help. It spilled over into ninety minutes instead of the usual sixty, and included much healing. Some time later I heard of its very positive effect, and this seemed really appropriate for this mini-death of an activity.

All that was left, therefore, was an openness to receiving one-day clients and possibly to facilitating short workshops. I felt rather as though the rug had been pulled out from under my feet, and wondered again about financial stability. However, trust, allowing and going with the Life Will had long been the belief I shared with my clients. Here I was, being pushed into the deep end myself. Thank goodness I can swim.

Those were the endings. What about the beginnings? It was New Year, a time when I really like to be on my own, to think both back and forward. This time I had decided not to make any New Year's resolutions. These always seemed to be very personality-oriented, and as perseverance has never been one of my strong qualities, they rarely remained effective for more than a few weeks. Sitting quietly that night, letting the old year run through my mind, seeing the new as a hope of new beginnings, I again asked 'the boys upstairs' for an idea. Instantly it was there. 'Go inside yourself and ask for the soul quality you most need to express during the coming year.' The word flashed into my mind: 'Sharing'. What a mundane suggestion! Nothing glamorous or inspiring, just sharing. Pain, joy, experience, age . . . I went in again and asked for a visualisation I could hold with the sharing concept. Instantly it too came. I saw the sea, a huge expanse, no land in sight, just water.

The first time it looked a bit grey and choppy, but over

the sea (was it because James Galway was playing at the time?) danced a lovely scatter of musical notes. And I understood. The sea was the 'now' in my life, and the music represented the sharing.

I use the visualisation rather as a barometer. How is the weather today? It varies enormously. Sometimes the sea is wild and stormy — the music may then be a booming foghorn, or it may be loud, harsh and unmelodious. Or there is a calm, quiet stretch of water, with the music a single, beautiful-sounding note. Contrarily, the same sea can also rest under a mournful minor requiem. Sharing the idea with a group I was surprised and delighted to find a full harmony sounding out above the water.

And almost at once the sharing started. The book I had written over a year previously began to shout for attention. I stalled at the thought of tackling and re-tackling publishers, but just then a visitor commented that a friend of hers had recently had a manuscript accepted by Findhorn Press. I ought to send mine there.

I immediately felt a connection, and after she had gone I sat down to describe how I *really* felt about the contents of the book. Unlike the formal blurb I had felt appropriate for other publishers, I talked about soul energy, spiritual need and the like. And also about the genuine affinity I felt this energy had with that of the Findhorn Community. As I posted it I remember thinking, "Either they'll understand, or they'll think I'm a real weirdie."

It was a delight to get a letter to say that they liked it, loved the title (*I Close My Eyes and See*) and felt they would be the ideal publishers. My reactions were interesting. Had it been accepted by the other publisher who had received it, and to whom I then would have had to say, "Sorry . . .", it would have been circulated quite widely in the large bookshops, and picked up by those interested in 'the spiritual'. This was fine, but at Findhorn, a spiritual community welcoming international visitors *seeking* the spiritual, the spread would be different, and to me felt much more satisfying.

With the contract signed, this second book was, so to speak, knocking on my door, and I can hear the third one lining up. I haven't spent time working out the connection, but all the death-in-life happenings undoubtedly freed me to this new birth-in-life.

It was not all roses, though. I had been so well. The relationship with Julian had either finished the ME episode, or sent it into a faraway remission. I thought about this. Why? How? And came to the conclusion that if healing must be directed to the whole person, then loving of the whole person must be a hugely strong healing resource. So it had been for me.

In practical terms it seems that the human immune system is weakened by grief and stress. Shortly after Christmas I got 'flu. It lasted about ten days, and then I was up and about again. But about a month later I suddenly got excruciating pain in my legs — just from the knees down. It was very variable. Sometimes stabbing pain stopped me in my tracks. Often whole areas went numb. In between, I just burned and tingled. Heat made it much worse. No more hot baths before bedtime. No thick duvet either. I hugged a hot water bottle to keep the top of me warm. Sitting with my legs up eased it a little, so my evenings were spent on the sofa. Driving any distance exacerbated the condition, and standing around was nearly impossible.

The first resource I used was radionics. But somehow I felt my practitioner was not tuning in to the right place. (Was I stopping this?) Intuitively I knew what it wasn't but couldn't pinpoint the cause, though there was obviously major disturbance of the physical nerves.

Finally, after two sleepless nights, I visited my GP. During this and further visits I had numerous blood tests, but they all came back negative. I was fascinated when a tuning fork held against my lower leg made absolutely no impression. I could not feel the vibration at all. Reflexes also vanished, and I was referred to a consultant. And still radionics made no impact. I went steadily through the maximum allowance of paracetamol, which took the edge off the constant pain.

The consultant merely suggested more tests and told me to come back in a month. I felt incredibly vulnerable and defenceless. No one seemed able to help. And my lifestyle of course closed in. It was painful to go to the shops, six miles away. I stopped for two coffee breaks each outing, just to sit down. I also had to completely cut out my social activities, including voluntary work. What next?

Finally it seemed that I had to stop thinking "Poor me" (and what a long time that had taken to sink in!) and either find help or just readjust to a different life mode. So I sat down and wrote a long letter to my homoeopath, telling him, as one must in homoeopathy, not only about my legs, but what was going on with all of me. By now, of course, Peter had been a steady support for me for a number of years. It was strange to think that he had originally come to me as a client, working through a two-day intensive. At that time he was still in general practice, but it was after visiting me that he started to train as a homoeopath, taking a six-month sabbatical to gain intensive experience in the final stages. I had recorded many personal tapes for him and had watched with delight as his spiritual awareness deepened. Then, in a truly wonderful way, it turned round and he became a support for me as well. Certainly, he is one of the people whose inner footsteps I hear very clearly.

He rang the next day and, homing in on the problem in his usual manner, suggested, "Reading between the lines, your letter was all about pain, life pain. And I think also it is about endings. Recently there have been so many endings in your life, some of them traumatic, and gradually you have gone down. That was the crucifixion. Now it's time for the resurrection. I *can* help you."

Usually, because of my sensitivity, he prescribed fairly low homoeopathic potencies. This time he used more drastic measures. I trusted him completely, which was as well, for the results from only two tiny tablets were quite frightening. The remedy was one for the nervous system, also for release of anger. I literally lost my balance for a few hours one day, the room swinging in vertigo. And of course, in my life I had lost my balance, and the pain of endings had moved into the endings of my limbs. As my sensitivities had increased I had already from practical experience become very aware of the close connection between mind, body and spirit. Any part could trigger the whole — towards the negative, towards the positive. Here was a huge illustration of this synthesis.

Two weeks later he gave me another remedy, this time more to do with shock, loss, grief and physical pain. Almost instantly it swung to my head. Intermittently my face went numb, my vision was affected and I had to 'stop' even more. Any concentration was impossible. But as another two weeks went by the headaches faded and I realised that some of the acute pain in my legs was gone. Change was continuing and in myself I found I was able to let go of at least some of the immediate and past problems of loss, which previously I had tended to worry at, dog-with-bone fashion.

My second visit to the consultant was more encouraging than the first. His conclusion that there was slight improvement in my condition was heartening. Not so heartening, however, was the letter to the insurance company stating that in his opinion I was not at this time fit to travel on holiday. He stated very honestly that he could not pin down the cause, and said he always found this situation disheartening. He still wanted further tests, and hoped that the very slow improvement would continue. The likely cause, having eliminated all others (including brain tumour which had not occurred to me at all!), might be post-infective nerve irritation. Back to the New Year 'flu — grief, shock, weakened immune system?

I felt there was a more holistic reason. Once again, I was being told to *stop*. ME had been quite different — long drawn out and exhausting, but not nearly so painfully crippling. What was it about? Letting go of pain, resentment, fear? Taking hold of trust, allowing, change without movement? The gift from this problem (definitely not asked for) was space. Sometimes it seemed like interminable space. And yet I had cleared a lot of it myself by voluntarily giving up most of my normal work load.

Was it coincidence that suddenly my general vulnerability was increased by a neighbour's unexpected attack on the boundaries of my land? I had always been able to park two cars below the terraced garden of my house. The new tenants next door blocked this, and when I mildly remonstrated, one of them appeared, shouting, at my front door. A phone call to my solicitor confirmed my 'rights', but I felt loath to maintain an aggressive argument. Remembering the Arcane School adage of 'Keep silence' I quietly maintained good relations with the neighbours. Now it seems that between us we can cool it. Whether it works or not, at least to some extent I have been able to let it go.

This brings to mind a life principle I have never managed, yet, to understand. I hold some negative attitude that I wish to change. I tell myself this, and I 'try', and nothing happens. The situation still annoys me. I still feel resentment. And it goes on and on, in spite of my wish. Then one day, the same or a similar situation occurs, and the negative attitude is GONE. I have done nothing different; it is still potentially maddening. Somewhere along the line I have let go. I can only think it must be some sort of marriage between will and allowing — and perhaps the ever-needed trust.

So what next? Where now? What is around the corner? I have absolutely no idea. And I believe that is the way it should be. I know what is mine at the moment. I have space. I have in many respects a huge freedom, few demands, little external responsibility. The temptation is to tell myself, "You're just a useless old woman who can no longer travel around sharing healing, leading workshops, offering constructive voluntary work help — *do*ing." Turn it all on its head and the answer flares out: "This is the time for *being*." And being is so much harder, I find, so much more responsibility, so much more demanding.

For while I may, albeit unintentionally, hoodwink other people, I can't fool myself. I honestly don't know a lot about being. Oh, I've talked about it quite a lot, shared it, thought about it. But this was in a comfortable part-time setting. Now, even if temporarily, I'm stuck with it full-time. Amusingly, the first question I ask myself is, "What can I *do* about it?" More difficult, but more accurate, is the question: "What can I *be* about it?"

The two must flow together at a deeper level. Like this. Energy must flow. Energy follows thought. Contemplation follows thought withheld. I have learned enough about energy to know that as I truly learn to be, then from this being, energy will not only be an outflow but will magnetise an inflow. Like attracts like. Inevitably I will share what I am learning and probably be approached by those who need to share this particular lesson with me.

This sharing has already started. One of my sons is an alcoholic. Through AA he is now learning about a Higher Power. He is also assimilating the idea of a God within (though emphatically not in that language). And we have started a long, deep correspondence. He asks me about my spiritual beliefs. I tell him some of what I have discovered, for me, and make it very clear that his path may be very different. Although in recovery, he is as yet unable to work, so he is in a state of *be*ing, different from and yet the same as mine.

One day I suggested, "Leave your antennae out and just pick up the spiritual in ordinary, ordinary things. You can pour a cup of tea for someone in a way that is totally spiritual. You can smile as you pass someone." He found this quite a new concept and passed it on to a lass in AA. She found it deeply helpful and actually stood up at the next meeting and talked about it. He was delighted. So was I.

Two letters later he described a concept that had just 'come to mind' for him, as an explanation of how his spirituality was developing. "Like a story," he said, "not a dream." I found it an amazing description of travel on the inner journey.

This was what he described. He said he likened himself to a small boy at Christmas time. He had been asking Santa for a tractor for months, and on Christmas morning he was handed a beautifully wrapped box, almost too big to hold. However, when he opened it, it wasn't a tractor at all, just a lot of bits and pieces. He was desperately disappointed, until his mother explained that the dozens of bits and pieces were the components with which the tractor could be built. The little boy wasn't sure about this; he wanted a tractor *now*. But once he got started, he became really engrossed in the making process.

It was difficult. Some of the bits were soft and nice to touch, some were hard. Some had round edges, some were sharp. He cut himself. But he persevered, and it began to take shape.

Then he got stuck and needed the instruction book. He found it, but it was in Japanese! So then he had to find someone who could understand the language and help him. His parents couldn't help him any more. And he did get help and went on building. As he got near the end he realised there were going to be a few pieces missing, and *these he would have to make for himself.*

What a discovery! It was immensely clear, right-side-of-the-brain symbolism — and from a hard-headed journalist, who was used to relying solely on the logic of words.

Sharing with him by letter was a little like sharing through letters related to the Arcane School. When my huge 'space' had become available, I had written to the School asking if there was anything I could do for them. To my surprise, horror, delight, I was asked if I would like to train to be a 'secretary'. This term describes senior students who begin to help those just starting the Arcane School work. It involves checking the meditation report, reading the set work and then writing helpfully, informatively, lovingly and impersonally with any comments. Criticism as such is disallowed.

I remembered well my beginning days and how much I looked forward to the secretary's letters. It almost struck me as a miracle that there was never a negative comment, just encouragement and sometimes useful suggestions — "Might it be . . . ?" "Do you think that . . . ?" — and bits of complementary information that just slotted in, increasing my understanding and also giving me confidence to plod on.

Could I do this? I made many rough copies of the first letters before, as a probationary secretary, I could return them to headquarters to be checked and approved before being passed on. It was difficult, interesting and very worthwhile.

In some ways it took me back to early Infant School teaching days. The four- and five-year-olds taught me so much as they looked at life through spectacles I had long discarded. It was sheer delight to go out into the playground with them, when the sun came out after a shower, and listen to their explanation of the ensuing steam. "Mind, it's smoke, it's dangerous." "No it isn't, it's the kettle, it'll burn you." Then, from one of the more sophisticated, "No, it's fog. Look it doesn't hurt." Concepts, concepts, concepts — wonder, joy, discovery.

These small children merited respect as well, just as in the bigger life outside school. I remember one rather insecure young teacher aghast when a four-year-old said to me (big white chief of the department), "You are so *stupid*." I wouldn't let her censure the child because, as I told her, "I *was* completely stupid from his point of view. I couldn't read his perfectly sensible writing."

Now I was dealing with adults, some of a good age, and frequently wearing different life spectacles. There were concepts to be shared, to be wondered about, sometimes to be discarded, but often, as with the infants, to keep, enriching one's own tentative discoveries.

Sharing in workshops requires the same qualities of respect and mutual discovery. I sent a list of themes to a group of eight women who have requested a workshop. Back came the reply, "Four of us want one theme, four another. Could you combine them?" Could I? I don't know yet. How does 'Why am I, where am I?' overlap with 'Harvest time'? I'm sure it will somehow. When I asked my local women's group for a possible single title, someone suggested simply 'Harvest me'.

Creativity continues, then, and there is space in my life now not just for consolidation but for further adventure. I wonder where, and why, and with whom? It feels a bit like setting sail again. My boat has a red sail and a 'trust' flag. In Meeting recently, as the doors stood open to the sun, and the wind hummed through the huge larch trees in the burial ground, a visitor stood up to minister and commented that we can hear the wind, but cannot see it. We can, however, see the results of its movement. Is the Spirit not like this too? And at once I pictured my little boat, way, way out on a still sea, with no wind at all, totally becalmed. I remembered the Breton fisherman's prayer: "Lord, the sea is so big, and my boat is so small."

This is the immediate 'now'. Tomorrow's 'now' may well be different. If it should be the same, then that is the place I AM. And so it should be.

My sharing year continues. The story I have shared here is only a life segment — or better, a tiny segment out of many lives. I believe this time I must have chosen to live a great deal of experience very quickly, and in concentrated form. So the ups have been high and shiny, and the lows sometimes a dark and sticky morass. I have tried to share with you some of the things I have learned as I have travelled. Your learning may be very different. But though we travel with different backpacks, different-sized boots, different heights, breadths, viewpoints, I suspect we are exploring many of the same themes and finding similar resolutions.

Resolution is the wrong word, though. This journey is about travelling, not yet about getting there; about persistence in direction, as the road swerves and changes and sometimes seems to lead us into a maze. For out of everything I have learned, I know now that the only safe certainty is uncertainty, and that security can only be found in the acceptance of change. You cannot hold something as dynamic as life in your hand. It needs to fly.

Trust, for me just now, is like a great bird. It can hover or swoop or soar, and on its back I can explore in safety. It may sometimes land on the water, where it does not need to flap or paddle, but just goes with the tide as the world turns round. And the waves break with a rippling song of "Don't try, just allow; don't try, just allow." And there is sound — my sound, your sound, life sound, and the great harmonies of LIFE I AM-ness singing. And that is NOW.

Always, trust offers exploration. The other day, in

meditation, I was focusing on the rainbow antahkarana bridge, linking my now with the Life Now. As I prepared to come back to humdrum daily life and mentally stepped off the rainbow, I saw that bits of light were sticking to my feet to share as I walked along. And I remembered that initial visualisation, in which I was told to spread coloured cats'-eyes around the world. It was similar, but subtly different. Then, I was being told to look and share what I saw. Now, I am told to keep walking in the Light, and that *is* the sharing.

And oh, I am glad you are walking with me!

Introducing Findhorn Press

Findhorn Press is the publishing business of the Findhorn Community which has grown around the Findhorn Foundation, co-founded in 1962 by Peter and Eileen Caddy and Dorothy Maclean. The first books originated from the early interest in Eileen's guidance over 20 years ago and Findhorn Press now publishes not only Eileen Caddy's books of guidance and inspirational material, but many other books, and it has also forged links with a number of like-minded authors and organisations.

For further information about the Findhorn Community and how to participate in its programmes please write to:

The Accommodation Secretary
Findhorn Foundation
Cluny Hill College
Forres IV36 0RD
Scotland
tel. +44 (0)1309-673655 fax +44 (0)1309 673113
e-mail reception@findhorn.org

For a complete catalogue, or for more information about Findhorn Press products, please contact:

Findhorn Press
The Park, Findhorn, Forres IV36 0TZ, Scotland
tel. +44 (0)1309-690582 fax +44 (0)1309-690036
e-mail thierry@findhorn.org
http://www.mcn.org/findhorn/press/ or
http://www.gaia.org/findhornpress/

Also available from Findhorn Press

• I Close My Eyes and See
Dorothy Lewis (author of *The Way Home*)

A treasury of beautiful and unique guided meditations and visualisations interspersed with the author's own warm, deeply touching and often humorous experiences on her own spiritual path as healer, teacher and workshop leader. Suggestions for using the visualisations with groups and sample workshop schedules are included.

Pbk   *176 pages*   *214x135mm*
£5.95/US$10.95/Can$15.50   *ISBN 1 899171 11 8*

• The Art of Psychic Protection
Judy Hall

A book of practical techniques and help for individuals or groups seeking to expand their consciousness. For those who meditate, use guided imagery or self-hypnosis tapes, for therapists and healers, for those who find excessive tiredness a problem, chances are that you need to protect yourselves with these tried and tested tools, some of which date back thousands of years whilst others belong to the 21st century. We protect ourselves in so many ways, we have tended to forget that psychic protection is a basic need.

Pbk   *144 pages*   *214x135mm*
£5.95/US$10.95/Can$15.50   *ISBN 1 899171 36 3*

• Playful Self-Discovery
David Earl Platts, Ph.D.

Designed especially for people who lead or take part in groups of any kind, this book describes a unique method of building trust in both new and established groups based on the Group Discovery Experience Week and workshop session presented for many years at the Findhorn Foundation. The session's light-hearted approach offers participants insight into their own personality and behaviour while fostering positive group dynamics, openness, cooperation and good will. This practical manual provides complete guidelines for preparing and presenting a full-length experiential session, including detailed instructions to 68 exercises and games, to help groups come together and function more effectively.

Pbk   *144 pages*   *214x135mm*
£5.95/US$10.95/Can$15.50   *ISBN 1 899171 06 1*

• The Path to Love is the Practice of Love

An Introduction to Spirituality with Self-Help Exercises
for Small Groups

Carol Riddell

Through the understanding and practice of spiritual principles, there
is the chance to transform daily life and find happiness in the service
of others. The teachings in this book can apply equally to all religions
as long as it is accepted that the essential principle of the cosmos is
love. The first section is channelled guidance, while the second part is
a series of exercises for ad hoc groups and workshops.

Pbk   *144 pages*   *214x135mm*
£5.95/US$10.95/Can$15.50   *ISBN 1 899171 20 7*

• Journeys Within

Source Book of Guided Meditations

Lisa Davis

Aimed at both individuals and groups needing help with guided meditations, this book gives the reader support in how to begin, conduct
and end meditations. It offers the opportunity to choose a topic from
a variety of subjects which can be recorded and used as required. For
anyone who is new to guided meditations or who has ever felt insecure or hesitant about leading them. It also gives opportunities for
experienced meditators to expand their repertoire, with topics such as
Tarot, Colour, Crystals and Healing.

Pbk   *144 pages*   *214x135mm*
£5.95/US$10.95/Can$15.50   *ISBN 1 899171 35 5*

• Choosing to Love

A Practical Guide for Bringing More Love into your Life

Eileen Caddy & David Earl Platts, Ph.D.

A book about the down-to-earth practicalities of exploring feelings,
attitudes, beliefs and past experiences which block us from loving.
Choosing to love is choosing to respect ourselves and others . . . Choosing to take down our inner barriers to love . . . Choosing to trust . . .
Choosing to take risks.

Pbk   *128 pages*   *214x135mm*
£5.95/US$10.95/Can$15.50   *ISBN 1 899171 90 9*

• Opening Doors Within

Eileen Caddy's most popular title — 365 pieces of guidance received during her meditations, one for each day of the year. They contain simple yet practical suggestions for living life with joy, inspiration and love. Translated into 12 languages, this treasure of a book is the perfect present for loved ones. Now available in both hardcover and paperback.

Hbk	*404 pages*	*£10.95/US$17.95/Can$24.95*
	ISBN 0 905249 66 6	
Pbk	*404 pages*	*£6.95/US$12.95/Can$17.95*
	ISBN 1 899171 68 2	

• The Kingdom Within

A Guide to the Spiritual Work of the Findhorn Community
Edited by Alex Walker, with contributions by David Spangler, William Bloom, Dorothy Maclean, Peter and Eileen Caddy and others.

A major work from and about the Findhorn Community. This collection of writings about the history, work, beliefs and practices of the Findhorn Foundation and its associated community of spiritual seekers offers a vision of hope, inspiration and encouragement to the world.

Pbk	*416 pages*	*214x135mm*
£8.95/US$14.95/Can$20.50		*ISBN 0 905249 99 2*

• Sights and Insights

A Guide to the Findhorn Foundation Community
Compiled by Cally and Harley Miller

This booklet is intended to give those of you who have only heard or read of this near-mystical place a clear and up-to-date picture of what the Community is like and of what there is to do and see here, as well as being a souvenir for those who have visited and love this place. Illustrated with line drawings of the most striking buildings in the Community, this guide will take you through the various developments of the last 34 years; it also places the Community in its surroundings with listings of local events, places of interest and nature walks.

Pbk	*48 pages*	*210x148mm*
£2.40/US$4/Can$5.50		*ISBN 1 899171 50 9*